Advance praise for *Some...*

Vicki Tapia's diary of the decline of her parents' lives due to Alzheimer's is a harrowing account of the gradual disintegration and ending of two lives in advanced age. It is also a daughter's loving memoir, a painstaking tale of the progression of dementia, with its sad, funny, mysterious, baffling, infuriating and frustrating series of incidents. At the end of each chapter Tapia summarizes what she has learned from her experience and how, with hindsight, it could have been improved, providing an excellent practical guide for the reader. This book is both a spellbinding modern tale and an invaluable resource.

Valerie Hemingway, author, *Running With the Bulls, My Life With the Hemingways*

Vicki Tapia's odyssey about caring for both parents with dementia is a testament to the resilience of the human spirit. One marvels at her ability to navigate through troubled waters, too often stirred up by well meaning yet misguided professionals. Her litany of lessons will help guide any family caregiver who may be in the same boat.

Daniel Kuhn, author, *Alzheimer's Early Stages: First Steps for Family, Friends and Caregivers*

I read the book over the weekend. I couldn't put it down! It many ways, it described universal experiences. I work in a memory care cottage plus my parents had dementia. I am anxious for my sister to read this book.

Faith Burrowes, RN and caretaker of dementia patients and adult daughter of an Alzheimer's patient

It's double indemnity as Mom and Dad descend into dementia hand-in-hand. The detailed personal story is interspersed with bite-sized bits of calming, reassuring advice, wisdom hard-won by Tapia during her time in the trenches. The author's gripping, detailed and sometimes funny account of her aged parents' simultaneous decline, and the repercussions for even far flung family, shows us definitively that "'Til death do you part" is not an injunction confined only to husbands and wives.

Eleanor Cooney, author, *My Mother's Descent into Alzheimer's DEATH IN SLOW MOTION*

This is a brave and powerful story. The thing that impresses me most about this is how Tapia doesn't back down from anything difficult, whether it's the grisly details of taking care of her parents' daily needs, or the emotional trauma that comes out of dealing with something this painful. I think Vicki does a terrific job of digging deep into those issues and telling this story with a frankness that makes it an important story.

Russell Rowland, Author, *In Open Spaces* and *High and Inside*

Vicki's book is wonderful. Such an easy read, and very compelling. I especially liked her honesty/transparency about her family relations. We all have dysfunctions in our families that we don't like to talk about...your observations add so much. This book is important for our generation as we care for, parent, and tend to our aging populations.

Dr. Douglas McBride, adult child of father with Alzheimer's

My dad had a cerebral hemorrhage yesterday. I told my daughter that I am so thankful that I had read your book (twice!) because from it I gained a lot of insight that will help me navigate through the tough decisions ahead.

> Diane Powers, Lactation Consultant, whose parents are both affected by dementia/Alzheimer's disease

Somebody Stole My Iron is a beautifully written narrative of the author's personal journey through the staggering maze of Dementia and Alzheimer's disease. She brings us with her from the beginning as she first discovers that something just doesn't seem quite right with, first her father and later her mother; who has become quite skilled in the art of camouflage and disguise. We the reader happily make the trip with her as the author leaps full force into this voyage, completely unaware of the depth of this disease. Once we begin, we soon find ourselves intertwined with every new development and transformation in the lives of this family. This warmly written book chronicles the life changing journey as she lovingly, bravely and relentlessly faces each and every challenge that this disease presents with both of her parents.

This is a 'must read', especially for those who may find themselves somewhere on this path as a loved one deals with any form of dementia.

> Lesli Gould, Lactation Consultant, Children's Clinic

I have spent most of the day reading this book, and found myself completely captivated. Vicki is a good writer, and her descriptions of your circumstances are so easy to visualize. ..I think that many who have experienced what she has could really relate to her experience!

Karel Horney, Executive Director of Adam's Camp, Denver, CO

I found the story riveting and could not stop reading it, even though I knew the outcome.

Rod Slater, Architect and son of mother with Alzheimer's, Auckland, NZ

Somebody Stole My Iron
A Family Memoir of Dementia

Vicki Tapia

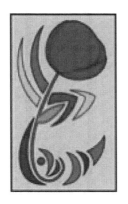

Praeclarus Press, LLC

www.PraeclarusPress.com

Praeclarus Press, LLC
2504 Sweetgum Lane
Amarillo, Texas 79124 USA
806-367-9950
www.PraeclarusPress.com

DISCLAIMER

The information contained in this publication is advisory only and is not intended to replace sound clinical judgment or individualized patient care. The author disclaims all warranties, whether expressed or implied, including any warranty as the quality, accuracy, safety, or suitability of this information for any particular purpose.

ISBN: 9781939807076

Cover Design: Ken Tackett

Acquisition & Development: Kathleen Kendall-Tackett

Copy Editing: Diana Cassar-Uhl

Layout & Design: Todd Rollison

Operations: Scott Sherwood

For Mom and Dad

According to the Alzheimer's Association (2012), one in eight older Americans has Alzheimer's disease. Alzheimer's disease is the sixth leading cause of death in the United States. Over 15 million Americans provide unpaid care for a person with Alzheimer's or other dementias.

TABLE OF CONTENTS

PREFACE

This is a story of one family's journey down the rabbit hole of dementia, focusing on Alzheimer's disease, from the perspective of the caregiver. I am the daughter and caregiver of two parents who each maneuvered, in their own way, through the devastating progression of dementia. My father, Harry Andersen, was diagnosed with dementia related to Parkinson's disease, and shortly thereafter, my 85-year-old mother, Trudy Blaine Andersen, with dementia's most common form, Alzheimer's disease.

Older patients, such as my father, who are diagnosed with Parkinson's disease are more at risk for developing Parkinson's-related dementia. Recent studies cite that more than 80 percent of people with Parkinson's disease over the age of 90 also suffer from dementia. Symptoms of Parkinson's-related dementia may include the inability to judge spatial relationships, attention problems, and visual hallucinations which are not typical of an Alzheimer's patient. My father was 90 years old when his Parkinson's disease was diagnosed, and the dementia component became apparent within a year of his diagnosis, when we realized his short-term memory was failing. While my father plays a part in this book, it is my mother who takes center stage, as we learned to cope (and sometimes failed to cope) with the progression of her disease.

Alzheimer's is a disease in which the brain slowly self-destructs from an accumulation of proteins running rampant inside and outside the neurons (nerve cells) of the brain. Researchers believe two proteins are involved: amyloid plaques and neurofibrillary tangles. The B-amyloid proteins produce tiny fibers (fibrils) that stick together to form the gooey amyloid plaques outside the neurons. The neurofibrillary tangles, primarily made up of tau protein, are twisted fibers that form inside the neurons.

It is normal for all of us to develop some plaques and tangles as we age, but a person suffering from Alzheimer's has a far greater accumulation of either or both. These plaques and tangles may somehow block the nerve cells' ability to communicate, thus disrupting the necessary action needed for cell survival. As brain cells die, the brain deteriorates, and actually shrinks.[1]

These plaques and tangles slowly and without apology replaced the normal cell structures in my mother's brain, and like a marshmallow held to the campfire flame, formed a sticky goo. There is currently no known way to stop the relentless march of this disintegration. Eventually the day arrived when my mother's brain appeared to be filled with more gooey marshmallows than brain cells, and I no longer recognized the woman I once called "Mom." I watched helplessly as the disease silently took away more and more of my mother, and she slowly but surely disappeared; first her mind, then her body.

Dementia can manifest in different ways, as evidenced by my parents' contrasting journeys. My mother's Alzheimer's was a journey of humiliation through the steady loss of control over her life. She anguished as she fought and clawed for command of the daily faculties she had so long taken for granted, attempting to climb up and out of the scary void. Heartbreakingly, she inescapably and gradually slipped away,

[1]*See Appendix A*

gathering herself in a dark place in the furthest corners of her mind, where no one else could venture.

My father seemed to deal with the changes as he had dealt with much of life—he simply accepted it. He rarely complained, and was compliant and easy to care for—a favorite of all his caregivers. His mind guilelessly glided away, as a balloon set free on a soft summer breeze. Watching my parents turn into people I no longer knew elicited many emotions within me, including sadness, frustration and helplessness. I often felt it was *me* entangled in the goo.

The journey did have its moments of black humor, almost always at the expense of my parents as their behavior often took a turn for the bizarre. This odyssey was confusing for all of us. Even reading and learning everything I could about dementia/Alzheimer's did not prepare me for all the behavioral changes that occurred as my parents declined into that fuzzy world where life seems to exist on a different plane; a place that none of us on *this* plane can truly understand. I sought to make the right choices in their care, but many instances presented uncharted territory for me and I often felt as if I was flying blind in my attempt to honor their requests while doing the "right" thing.

Dementia is a disease of confusion for the person who suffers from it, as life becomes a series of never-ending daily challenges. These challenges begin with something so simple as waking up in the morning and getting out of bed, and end when a caregiver tucks them back into that same bed, much as if they were small children. Every task that we, who exist in the "normal" cognitive world take for granted eventually becomes an indecipherable maze for the person suffering from dementia.

For me, the path was tangled with both heartbreak and personal growth. I have never aspired to keep company with grief and despair, but they were often my companions. However, I also learned how to reach into the depths of my inner self and discover more hidden compassion and understanding with each passing day.

What follows is our story, based on my memories and perceptions through a difficult time of change, upheaval, and growth. It is a story of holding on, and ultimately, of learning how to let go.

AUTHOR'S NOTE

This memoir is designed to be more than just a story of my experience. My goal is to ease the burden for you, the reader, as you undertake the journey with your loved one down the often difficult road of dementia. I was not prepared for this journey, and many lessons I learned after the fact--that is, I learned them "the hard way." In hindsight, there are things I would have done differently, and perhaps better had I had some sort of road map.

In the hopes of lightening your load as you wind your way down the path of similarly challenging experiences and situations, I have shared my learned lessons with you at the end of many chapters. My goal is to provide a base from which you can further call upon your ability to accept, understand, and feel compassion while you maneuver through the many facets of dementia. Part One recalls my memories as our family edged closer and closer to the uncharted territory of my mother's odyssey through Alzheimer's. In Part Two, the disease continues to unfold in "real time."

I would like to acknowledge and offer a special thanks to my assistant editor and daughter, Jill Chiasson, without whose never-failing encouragement and superior editing skills this book would still be a collection of words in my computer files. I thank author Russ Rowland, who gave me direction and helped draw out more details to shape the book. I am grateful for family members Megan Nyquist, Kyle and Kylee Bodley, who put the finishing touches on the editing. I'd also like to recognize and thank my son-in-law, Blake Nyquist, who designed my superb website, and my stepson, Nicholas Tapia, whose vision helped create the video trailer and audio excerpts on my website (www.SomebodyStoleMyIron.com). This was, in some ways, truly a family endeavor!

Over the past five years, there have been others along the way, who offered helpful suggestions and edits, including Kitty Cutting, Karen Jarussi, Karel Horney, Kathie Shandera, Rod Slater and my husband, Lionel, to whom I offer my sincere appreciation. Thanks also to Diane Powers, who ignited the spark to write this memoir when she repeatedly said to me, "you are writing this down, aren't you?" whenever I shared a story about my parents' journey.

Names of some people and places have been changed to protect privacy. The conversations in this memoir were written after the fact, but are as true to the actual conversations as I remember them.

PART ONE

London Bridge is Falling Down

ONE
Endings and Beginnings

"Mom, what should I do with this?"

I look across the cluttered room from where I am knee deep in items, sorting, absently noting the sunlight streaming through the lone window, momentarily distracted by the dust motes dancing in the air. There stands my daughter, Jill, framed by the sunlight, holding up a slightly tarnished and dented wastebasket amidst the piles of clothing, bedding, knick-knacks, pillows, stuffed animals, and other randomly piled personal effects.

That brass wastebasket used to be in the condo bedroom, right next to Mom's night table, I remember, *when it didn't have a dent or look like someone had sat on it.* I hear myself answer my daughter in a business-like voice, "Oh, put it with the rest of the stuff going to Charity Services." She adds it to one of the rapidly growing mounds of discarded belongings on the floor of my mother's room at the assisted-living facility.

I have disconnected my heart from my brain this afternoon, as I mechanically sort through what is left of my mother's life. She has no further use for anything in this room. I glance again at the wastebasket now sitting forlornly on top of a blanket. Memories flood in without my permission and I am taken back, to a different time and place. How could we all have missed the signs? In hindsight, reflecting on six long years ago, it is hard to imagine missing them, because they were there. It all started with a computer.

"Grandma Trudy, I am so excited; I am getting a new computer!" my vivacious niece, Katie, exclaimed over the phone from her apartment in Portland, Oregon.

"That's wonderful," Mom enthusiastically agreed.

"Yeah, and the reason I'm calling is because I thought maybe you'd like my old computer."

"Well, honey, I don't know. I'm not sure at this stage of the game we'd even be able to figure out how to use it."

"Oh, Grandma, I really think you could learn! We could e-mail each other and besides that, there are computer games already downloaded on it that I just know Grandpa Harry would love to play!"

By the end of the conversation, Katie had convinced her skeptical Grandma Trudy to give the computer a try. My niece boxed up her computer monitor, hard drive, and software, and within a week, UPS delivered two large, well-padded boxes to my parents, who lived approximately 1,000 miles east of Portland. They were about to join the digital age.

Word quickly spread through the family grapevine that Grandma and Grandpa were the recipients of Katie's old computer. Because neither my brother Jack, myself, nor any of their five grandchildren lived nearby, everyone concurred that the computer was a brilliant idea, and were excited to begin sending computer-scanned pictures of our families, and trading e-mails. My parents were bright people, and we also recognized that learning how to operate a computer would be good "brain food" for them.

My mother, who was in her early 80s at the time, was most interested in learning how to send e-mails, and my father, in his late 80s, was content to watch the "magic" happen on the screen, although he eventually did learn to play a few easy computer games, like solitaire. Mom was never terribly technologically proficient, but most of the time, she managed to make the computer work for her. For a while, family members were able to e-mail back and forth with them, although not as often as anyone had anticipated.

As time went on, it seemed Mom was having more and more difficulty with the computer, as one glitch after another began to occur.

Regardless of e-mail, we typically talked on the phone several times a week, and our conversations started to take on a familiar theme:

"Hi, Mom! What's new?"

"Well, honey, that darn computer is acting up again. I just can't make it go. I called the Internet people, and they sent that same nice young man over again, and as usual, it seemed to work fine for him. He went over everything another time for me. Maybe I'm just too stupid to work a computer."

"Oh, of course not, Mom. Maybe we can go over it all again when I come to visit next weekend?" I lived in Coulson, two hours west of where they lived in Nelson City, and visited weekends as often as my schedule would allow.

"Okay, you sure can try, but I just think I'm getting too old for this sort of thing."

Over the course of the next year, several members of our family sat down at the computer with her when we visited to give her yet another "tutorial." At the moment of instruction, she nodded her head with seemingly complete understanding, and took copious notes. In retrospect, we didn't realize how well developed her acting skills had become. We also wrote down notes, and I even drew pictures for her, to help her remember the process. Ultimately, it seemed the computer became so littered with yellow sticky notes we could barely see the screen! None of our tutorials and notes seemed to help. No matter how patiently we repeated the information, or how many pictures we drew, every time we left her house, her ability to operate the computer walked out the door with us.

TWO
Celebrating 90 Springs

My mom, Trudy Blaine Andersen, had lived in Nelson City, Montana her entire life, and my dad, Harry, since he was a teen. They grew up with Nelson City during the 20th century, watching it grow from a small "cow town" in the early part of the century through the Depression and onward. Harry Andersen helped steer Nelson City into the modern world in his own way as the town's mayor from 1957-1969. He was also a grocer, starting in the business as a teen, and eventually operating his own corner grocery store for more than 40 years. To this day, I meet people whose eyes brighten when they hear who my father was. They all delight in sharing how they frequented his store as a child, with fond memories of his "penny" candy. He doted on these children, giving them each a small brown paper bag, and in exchange for their often-sticky pennies, he watched them fill up their bags with sumptuous treats.

The advent of supermarkets spelled the demise of small corner groceries, and by 1978, when Dad was 65, the time was ripe to retire. After retirement, Mom and Dad stayed active in the community through their church and many different volunteer organizations. In their small town, my parents knew everyone, and everyone knew them. They made it clear to all of the family members over the years that they expected not only to continue *living* in Nelson City, but they planned to die there as well. This small community had been their social epicenter for more than three-quarters of a century, and they had no desire to ever leave.

In May of 2003, my father celebrated the 90th anniversary of his birth with a family reunion weekend in Nelson City.

Jack and I invited all the relatives to attend and honor our father on his big day. On the appointed weekend, one by one, we breezed in from various parts of the country to celebrate the momentous event. We gathered at our parents' condo on a sunny and warm Saturday morning. Their living room was filled with the chatter and chaos of a family reunion, along with a couple of fragrant bouquets of spring flowers from relatives unable to attend. Dad, with his usual calm, sat in his recliner smiling, soaking up all this family warmth like rays of sunshine. On the other hand, instead of enjoying us being together, Mom worried about each of us tracking dirt onto their carpet. We took our shoes off.

My nieces, Deanna and Katie, who live on the west coast, were surprise guests. After the rest of us were already gathered, we planned the "surprise arrival" so that the doorbell rang twice, once for each granddaughter and separated by a few minutes, so as not to cause too much excitement for Dad and Mom all at once. Katie was the first to ring the doorbell. Mom answered the door, "Oh my goodness! Look who is here; it's Katie!" Katie walked into the living room to greet and hug her Grandpa. "Hello Grandpa! Happy Birthday!"

"Well, Katie! What a surprise!" he said, returning the hug with obvious pleasure.

After a few minutes the doorbell rang again.

"Now, who could that be?" asked my mother as she hurried across the room. There in the doorway stood Deanna.

My mother, looking a bit confused, stared at her granddaughter and said, "Who are you?"

Deanna's face fell. The rest of us looked on in shocked disbelief. "Who am I? Why, I am Deanna, your granddaughter," she replied in a perplexed and somewhat shaky voice.

It was another clue that we somehow brushed off, attributing it to the stress of taking care of Dad and the commotion of having so many visitors all at once. Looking back, it is now obvious to me that our minds are well-tuned to rationalizing strange events or behavior in our attempt to normalize life.

THREE

Another of Life's Nose-Dives

Spring melted into summer, and concern for Mom took a back seat to Dad, as his coordination took an unexpected and sudden decline.

"Vicki, I don't know what I am going to do with your dad," Mom complained one day, during one of our frequent phone calls. "He's become just plain clumsy."

"Harry, for crying out loud, pick up your feet!" In my mind I could hear Mom hollering at my once-spry and agile Dad as he stumbled, barely escaping falling flat on his face on the sidewalk as they took their daily walk around the neighborhood.

Lionel, my husband, and I sensed it was more than simple clumsiness.

"Oh Vicki, your dad (*she always referred to him as "your dad," like he was only family to me, not her*) fell on the sidewalk yesterday, and landed on his shoulder and face. He broke his glasses, and you should see his black eye! He's limping around today because, when he fell, he also banged up his knee. I don't think we are going to be able to continue taking walks. He insists he's okay, but I'm not so sure ... "

Lionel, a physician, had mentioned to me more than once that Dad seemed to walk with an erratic gait—he was concerned it might be Parkinson's disease. I always thought a person with Parkinson's disease had visible shakiness, with head bobbing and hands quivering, but learned that this is not always so. Mom was also concerned, so she didn't need much encouragement to set up a doctor's appointment for Dad.

"Hi Vicki. Well, the doctor says your Dad has Parkinson's disease." My husband's suspicions were thus confirmed. I don't know how Dad felt about the diagnosis, as he never talked about it with us.

My dad's overall walking ability slowly began to falter, and although he was still able to walk mostly unassisted, my parents' days of strolling around their neighborhood were numbered. These walks became stressful for Mom, as Dad's lack of balance resulted in more tumbles.

"Your Dad is going to be the death of me yet!" Mom exclaimed to me on the telephone. "He tripped walking up the porch steps today, and started to fall, but luckily I caught him, so he didn't hurt himself, but he scared the wits out of me!" she said. "This is what happens when he doesn't mind me and use his cane. I'm just going to start leaving him home when I go out to the store and church. We'll see how he likes that!" she fumed.

In all his assorted spills, there were no broken bones, but there were ample bruises, skinned elbows and knees, a couple of black eyes, plus another broken pair of eyeglasses. In spite of this, my dad did not give up, and although he spent less time walking, he continued to embrace living, focusing his attention on activities that could be done from the comfort of his armchair, like crossword puzzles, reading, or watching television. Dad seemed to innately know the secret of contentment.

He relied more and more on Mom's help in getting out of chairs or bed. Even though she was rather petite at 5' 4", Mom seemed to harbor an inner strength, often supporting my father's 5' 9" 140-pound frame. Nevertheless, one of my larger concerns at the time was that he would end up pulling Mom down—or even worse, falling on her. As the spring of 2004 approached, he began walking less and less, and when he did, he usually "minded" his wife, using a cane to steady himself. A quiet man, Dad appeared to take these new developments in stride; I never heard him utter one word of complaint or despair.

Parkinson's disease was not his only health concern. He also had a slow-growing prostate cancer, which resulted in his awakening several times a night with the urge to urinate. Within a few months of his Parkinson's diagnosis, he could no longer make his way to the toilet without my mother's help. This meant she was getting less sleep, and having more trouble coping with the situation. Dad could always grab ample naptime during the day since he spent most of his waking time sitting in his plush recliner, maneuvering to the dining room table to eat, and then back to the chair for a nap. Mom, on the other hand, was never much for daytime naps and just became more stressed, run down, and sleep-deprived.

Mom was also coping with intensifying rheumatoid arthritis, which seemed more pronounced each time I visited. Bent and misshapen, the fingers on her right hand reminded me of gnarled tree roots, knotted and growing at seemingly unnatural angles. Worse yet was the way her right knee twisted sideways as she walked. She was in constant pain, which did nothing to help her already irascible mood. Her doctor had been unable to provide a pain medication that brought relief, so she simply lived with the pain, day after day, and continued to suffer from sleep deprivation caused by Dad's frequent nightly needs. Despite this, however, my parents were stubbornly of the mind that they "did not need any help," and all suggestions of home health care were abruptly dismissed.

FOUR
Something is "Off"

One day in that spring of 2004, my college-aged children, Jill and Kyle, were home on a school break. I took a vacation day from my part-time job as a lactation consultant so the three of us could drive to Nelson City to visit for the day. Mom and Dad were happy to see the three of us arrive that morning, as we brought some welcome diversity to their otherwise mundane days. Dad held court in his armchair while Mom scurried about making sure everyone tasted one of her cookies, slightly burned—an incongruous result for someone my kids always considered the "queen of cookie-makers."

"Kyle, have another cookie."

"Um, sure Grandma." We all did our best to be polite. We had a chance to catch up on family news, and before we knew it, it was time for lunch. We moved from their cozy living room into the kitchen/dining area.

"Kyle, can you help Grandpa get to the table?" my mom asked her grandson. "Put his bib on, and be sure you put him in the chair over the plastic floor mat," she instructed him. "He is so sloppy when he eats," she continued, talking about him as if he wasn't in the room. She didn't want any crumbs on her carpeting. *How does she manage this on her own*, I wondered, as I watched Kyle guide his unsteady grandpa into the dining room chair. Grandpa said nary a word. After nearly 70 years of marriage, he was used to her belittling ways.

"There is some sliced turkey meat for sandwiches in the refrigerator, especially for you," Mom stated, as she took the twist tie off a loaf of bread. "Jill, will you pull out some plates for me? This darn arthritis makes it a little hard to reach up in the cupboard and take out the plates."

Sandwich in hand, Kyle walked over to the refrigerator, reached in and took the clear plastic milk carton out of the refrigerator to pour himself a glass of milk. He suddenly looked over to me with questioning eyes, and when I followed his eyes to the milk carton, I saw what he had noticed. There was green mold growing on the inside of the carton. *Uh oh, this is not good.* Kyle obviously wasn't sure what to do next, and was looking to me to say something.

"Gosh, Mom, maybe that milk is past its prime," I cautiously ventured while Kyle carefully poured it down the drain. My mind was racing. *What is going on here?* This was so unlike my mother, who had always been a most meticulous housekeeper. She looked confused, gave me a sharp look, and responded defensively, "Well, it wasn't that way earlier. It tasted just fine at breakfast." This response did not alleviate my fear that something was amiss.

The five of us sat around their dining table and ate a rather silent lunch, Kyle and I knowing we had insulted her by inferring that she kept moldy milk in her refrigerator. As I cleaned up the dishes, I thought to myself, *what is that smell?* I picked up her dishcloth and was overcome by a noxious stench. Knowing that I was already walking on thin ice from the milk incident, I quietly walked down the hall and put the dishcloth in the laundry room. Surreptitiously, I retrieved a clean cloth from the drawer. I later learned this action did *not* go unnoticed by my mother. The rest of the visit was uneventful, meaning none of us got into any further "trouble" with Mom, and by late afternoon we said our goodbyes and drove back to Coulson.

"Mom, I don't see how they can continue living on their own," Jill stated on our drive back. We all agreed the situation could not be expected to improve, but were unsure when the tipping point might be with respect to their stubbornness at refusing outside help. The visit left us all unsettled.

Several days later, I was sitting on my couch reading when the phone rang. It was Mom. She had called to chastise me for our comments about her housekeeping abilities.

"How dare you say those things to me! I know you think I am a filthy housekeeper. I don't do anything right." She got right to the point of her call, and her tirade went on and on.

I was confused, hurt, and bewildered by her outburst. "Mom, calm down. We were only concerned that the moldy milk might make you ill."

"Well, I know you think I'm dirty. I *saw* you move my dishcloth to the laundry room, and I want to know what you were up to! You think you're so sneaky. I'm just dumb and filthy." Her anger triggered a sense of panic inside me, as I suddenly became five years old again, terrified I was in trouble and might be slapped if I talked back.

I snapped back to reality, and in a calm voice attempted to reason, "Mom, Mom, Mom. Listen to me. I'm sorry you feel this way. I didn't do this to upset you, only to help you." How little I understood at the time and how poorly I handled the situation as she went on to berate and scold me. The conversation ended with me in tears, actually hanging up on her in the middle of her ranting and raving. *What was happening? Who was this woman?*

Only a few minutes later she called back and apologized, as did I for giving her the impression she was a "filthy" housekeeper. We never spoke of it again.

Now, looking back, the real issue was that we still didn't "get it." We attributed her behavior to the stress she was experiencing in light of my father's declining health. It seems nothing short of miraculous that my parents were able to cope and live on their own for as long as they did. This ability is a testament to their generation's "can-do" mentality and self-sufficiency.

Lessons Learned

if something seems "off," consider the possibility that it is more than simple stress or "old age." Seek information and guidance by steering your loved one to his/her health care professional (HCP) for a checkup and evaluation.

Start honing your patience. You will need an abundance of it.

Pre-Diagnosis

Have Durable Power of Attorney in place long before it is needed for legal concerns and a HIPAA release for health care concerns. I was very fortunate that my parents had planned ahead, and given my brother and me Durable Power of Attorney years before they were actually needed, so I was later able to interface directly with their HCP (had I not had this power of attorney, my parent's healthcare information would have been off-limits to me because of privacy laws). If you are unable to convince your loved one to sign a Durable Power of Attorney, perhaps his/her HCP can be called upon to interface for you in this regard.

If you're unable to persuade your loved one to grant you or another family member Durable Power of Attorney, you may find it necessary to go to court and get a conservatorship. Generally, this can be accomplished in an expedited manner to deal with most emergencies. For more information, contact the National Academy of Elder Law Attorneys through their website at http://www.naela.org/.

FIVE
Diagnosis

Somehow, Mom and Dad managed to continue their routine: grocery shopping on the same day each week, collecting their mail each day from their post office box, and attending Sunday church. In addition, Dad's doctor wrote orders for home health care to provide physical therapy in hopes of keeping him mobile for as long as possible. Thank goodness that was acceptable "help" to the two of them.

My mother's memory issues continued to concern me.

"Hi Vicki. Well, we didn't find the cat."

"What cat? Mom, you don't have a cat."

Ignoring me, she went on, "I went to the grocery store today, but the vegetables were in terrible condition. It was the neighbor's cat," she added, as an apparent afterthought.

"How are you doing, Mom? How is Dad sleeping?"

"I only slept a couple of hours last night as your Dad got me up four or five times to go to the bathroom. Honestly, I don't know what I'm going to do with him. I think he does it on purpose to keep me from sleeping. We're doing fine, though," as if this last comment would reassure me.

She continued, "That nice boy from the hospital came over yesterday and showed your dad some exercises he could do to help him walk better."

"That's great, Mom. What does Dad say about it? Does he think it's helping?"

"Oh, you know your dad, Vicki, he never says much. He did everything the boy told him to do, so I think maybe he will start walking better now, if I make him practice what the boy taught him."

Well, we can always hope, I thought to myself.

"So, Mom, what's for dinner tonight?"

"Oh, I need to go take him to the bathroom. He thinks he can get up from his chair by himself, and he can't. Bye." Click.

Telephone conversations were often odd and ended abruptly, which gave me the feeling I wasn't hearing the full story. I wasn't sure if she was fearful of the family having some sort of intervention and moving Dad, or her, or both of them, to an assisted-living/nursing home, or whether she simply couldn't remember the answers to my questions. I wondered what was going on in her mind during these conversations. She *did* want to let me know she and Dad were doing "just fine," even though he had gotten her up numerous times the previous night to help him to the bathroom. I wasn't sure whether the memory issues were simply sleep deprivation, normal aging, or something else. My intuition told me it might be something else, and eventually I made a call to her primary care giver, a nurse practitioner, and requested she evaluate Mom. Amazingly, when I approached Mom about making a visit to her nurse practitioner, she didn't argue.

This evaluation became a turning point for our family. Part of me wanted to know the truth, but another part wanted to stay within the comfortable confines of denial. I was fearful that it might be Alzheimer's disease, or some other type of dementia. I was also confused as to the difference between the two. In my search for answers, I learned that Alzheimer's is one of about 70 different types of dementia and, a diagnosis of Alzheimer's while a patient is still living has a 90 percent accuracy rate.[2]

[2] *See Appendix B.*

A person suffering from Alzheimer's has very specific brain abnormalities, although in a typical medical practice, physicians can't "see" these microscopic brain anomalies. Since there is no clear-cut method of evaluating someone for Alzheimer's disease, physicians evaluate through a physical exam, diagnostic tests, a neurological exam, and mental status test. Brain imaging with MRI or CT scans may be used, but generally only to detect tumors, evidence of strokes, or head trauma. At the time of my mother's diagnosis in 2004, the nurse practitioner in her small community did not do any scans, but used one of the most common assessment tests of mental function called the Mini Mental State Examination (MMSE).[3] This exam looks at difficulties with memory and helps diagnose varying degrees of dementia, so it is not simply a test for Alzheimer's.

Mom's nurse practitioner called me with the news, "A score of less than 22 is considered abnormal. Your mother scored 18."

"What does that mean, exactly?" I asked.

"Well, her prognosis isn't good. She can now be classified as suffering from moderate Alzheimer's disease."

In hearing this diagnosis, it was like a light flickered on inside my head—things were suddenly so much clearer. On my most recent visit to my parents' house, Mom announced, "There are some things in my kitchen drawers, and I don't know why I have them." She led me into the kitchen, opened one of the drawers where cooking gadgets were kept, and pointed to some eggbeaters, saying, "What in the world are these for?" The symptoms are obvious to me now, but at the time, I again used the fact that she must be overwhelmed caring for Dad as an excuse for her confusion.

---

[3] *See Appendix C for scoring information on the MMSE.*

My bright, perfectionist mother had Alzheimer's. In years gone by, multi-tasking had been easy for my mother, as she juggled several part-time jobs, both paid and volunteer, with no difficulty. She was the consummate housekeeper, who prided herself on a clutter-free home, and was a meticulous dresser. She was an "idea person" who could be called upon to solve any number of household dilemmas, and I often thought of her as my own private Heloise. How could she have this awful disease?

The *actual* diagnosis of Alzheimer's vs. the *possibility* of Alzheimer's proved to be much more difficult to wrap my mind around. Prior to her diagnosis, I held onto hope that there was a medicine that could "fix" her and return her to her former self, the mother I knew. With the diagnosis, a door slammed shut. There is no cure for Alzheimer's yet, only a downward spiral of the mind as the disease progresses, sometimes quickly and sometimes over many, many years— either way resulting in death.

I had done some research and learned that while there was no cure for this disease, there is a medication called Aricept that will alleviate the symptoms for some people.[4] In clinical trials, Aricept had been shown to delay Alzheimer's symptoms from worsening for a period of up to a year for about 50 percent of the Alzheimer's patients who had taken it, and these beneficial effects have lasted even longer for some.

---

[4] *Aricept is a type of Cholinesterase inhibitor that prevents the breakdown of acetylcholine. Acetylcholine is a "chemical messenger" that carries neural messages between the brain's nerve cells, and is important for memory and learning.*

Mom began taking Aricept in August of 2004, as prescribed by her nurse practitioner. Our hope was that this medication would extend Mom's ability to remain independent. In addition to Aricept, she was prescribed an antidepressant for her low mood. This marked the beginning of her pill odyssey.

The nurse practitioner advised Mom that a home health care person would be stopping by regularly to help set up her medications, which eased *my* mind. Thankfully, when her nurse practitioner announced this arrangement, Mom didn't argue. From two hours' drive away, I was very appreciative of this service. At the same time, I knew this situation couldn't go on indefinitely. Changes loomed on the horizon.

How far could I go in pushing my parents to make changes when their safety was involved? When would they begin to accuse me of overstepping my boundaries and of being disrespectful? I felt like a novice tightrope walker, destined to fall. Their safety was still my chief concern, and I knew that in the not-too-distant future, intervention would be necessary; I also knew that they would not take it well. I suspect no one likes to be told they can no longer live on his or her own. By nature I'm a non-confrontational person, so instead of dealing with the issue, I pushed it into a far corner of my mind.

During this time my dad's memory was also failing, but it was less apparent because he wasn't a conversationalist. He rarely ever spoke on the telephone, so my awareness of his memory loss was minimal. Short-term memory loss is often a component of Parkinson's disease in the elderly, so I wasn't surprised when I did become aware of his loss. I now realize it's easier for quiet people to conceal such disabilities.

Lessons Learned

When it becomes evident that more care or medication might be needed, try to enlist the assistance of your loved one's health care provider (HCP). Mom was more receptive and accepting of the idea of taking medication to aid her conditions (depression and memory loss) when it was suggested by her HCP. When I suggested to Mom and Dad they have someone from home health care come into their home to help them, it was met with resistance, but when their HCP suggested it, they readily agreed. It was also helpful that I was able to speak with the HCP before Mom's appointment to fill in the information gaps that might arise when she met with Mom.

I would recommend learning as much as possible about dementia if a loved one is diagnosed with Alzheimer's, or any other form of dementia. It will help brace you for the changes that loom ahead. I found that our town's local senior resource center as well as our Alzheimer's Association chapter office were filled with useful medical information describing dementia/Alzheimer's disease, including movie documentaries, books and brochures, as well as a sympathetic ear to offer support and encouragement. The Alzheimer's Association Green-Field Library in Chicago, the largest Alzheimer's (and dementia) library and recourse center in the U.S., is another valuable resource. This library houses more than 5,000 books, journals and CDs, along with librarians to help you. Visit this virtual library on the web at http://www.alz.org/library/index.asp.

SIX
Sibling MIA

During the summer of 2004, the last time my parents were together in their condo, my brother Jack and his wife Rhoda traveled the 900 miles from their home for a visit. This would be the last time they visited Mom and Dad in their home in Nelson City. Although they didn't share their concern with me, Jack and Rhoda must have had some apprehension about Mom and Dad's behavior as Mom related to me later that Jack and Rhoda had asked for, and taken, Dad's diamond ring and his extensive silver coin collection before they left. When Mom shared this information with me, and didn't seem bothered about it, I decided there was no point even mentioning she and Dad had previously told me, and put in writing, that part of the silver coin collection would be left to me. This incident added to my growing irritation with my brother for what seemed to me a lack of empathy and involvement in our parents' lives.

This was the summer it became apparent that I would essentially be the sole caregiver of my parents, as my brother elected to be neither helpful nor involved. Others who have traveled the same path with their parents tell me that if there's a daughter in the family to take the role of "chief" caregiver, sons are typically content to remain safely in the background. While this proved to be the case in our family, I also realize proximity can play a part.

After Jack and Rhoda's visit that summer, they visited Mom and Dad twice over the next three years for one or two-day visits, and then returned for our mother's funeral. Telephone conversations were as close as they wished to be to the situation. I felt the burden that an only child, or others in a similar situation, can understand as their parents' health starts to fail. This added stress to my life, but, my parents had always been there for me. They showed up to help when my children were born, traveled to my home to care for our children so my husband and I were able to have getaways, and were generous financially if a particular need arose. They were especially supportive when I went through a divorce. They both sustained me emotionally and helped me financially, so I remained determined to do all I could to help *them* now, with the same love and care that they had always shown me.

Lesson Learned

"It is what it is." If you find yourself as the primary family caregiver beginning this journey unsupported by your sibling(s), enlist the help of your spouse, if you have one, or find another supportive relative or friend to stand by your side. If there is not a friend who can provide adequate support for you, join a local support group for families of people with memory loss. If there is no local group, find an online support group. Do not go through this difficult experience alone without a support network of some type, as it will begin to take its toll on *your* mental health.

SEVEN
Broken Hips, Broken Dreams

After Jack and Rhoda returned to their home, Jack began regularly calling our mother in an attempt to convince her to rearrange beneficiaries in her will. Mom told me that he felt the inheritance was not equitable. Mom assured him that she and Dad had spent a great deal of time making sure that it *was* equitable. As the calls continued, she began to feel pressured by him, which made her very angry. She also developed a skin condition, which she nervously scratched until she bled.

"Vicki, your brother won't leave me alone! He calls here all the time wanting me to put his name on the stock certificates that are in your name. I am going to take his name off of everything," she threatened, and began to call him by any number of unbecoming names.

After listening to these tirades for several weeks, it finally occurred to me to call my brother, and ask him to stop what I felt amounted to harassment.

"Jack, your phone calls are terribly upsetting to Mom. She calls me crying after every time you call her. She scratches her back until it bleeds. Will you please STOP?" I begged him. The only way he agreed to stop the phone calls was if I signed and notarized a document saying any funds left after our parents' demise would be split jointly between us. Although I could not understand his feelings that I might somehow try and cheat him, I didn't hesitate to do what he demanded in order to stop the torment for our mother, even as Lionel shook his head in disgust over the whole situation.

As summer waned, Mom continued to be worn down by both lack of sleep and caring for Dad, who was becoming more dependent by the week. He now needed a walker to navigate his way around the condo.

"Mom, what would you think of hiring someone to give you a hand with housework or grocery shopping?" Whenever I tried to suggest she enlist this type of help, she responded curtly with some variation of, "No, thanks. I am perfectly capable of doing it on my own. I have my own way of doing things, and there isn't anyone who would be able to do it the way I want it done."

During our many phone conversations, I continued to voice my concerns and also urged another option—for her to consider assisted living for my father, or for both of them. I wanted Mom to have control over decisions that affected her life, so when she continued to fiercely resist the idea of a helper with all the stubbornness she could muster, I chose not to argue. I was completely astonished when she called one day towards the end of August with some startling news, proving she was definitely still in control.

"Well, I did it," she proudly stated.

"Did what, Mom?"

"Took your dad to Winterhaven Manor. I went out there, and asked them if they would keep him for ten days in respite care. I'll bring him home in ten days. They told me that after that, whenever I want to, it is okay to bring him back out for daily care."

I was so shocked, and it took me a few seconds to recover and squeak out, "Really? Why? What happened? Is he okay? Are you okay?" She had been so adamant in all our conversations about *never* taking him to a nursing home.

"Last night was the last straw!" She explained. "My arthritis was acting up, and as I tried to help him up out of his chair to grab his walker, he slipped out of my grip, fell and knocked over his walker." After pausing, she went on, " ... which pushed it into me, and I toppled into a heap on top of him. I can't go on like this." Her strong voice suddenly disintegrated into sobs. My mom doesn't cry easily.

I quickly recovered and said, "Oh, Mom, I am so sorry! So sorry..." my voice drifted off. "For your sake," I managed, after I found my voice, "that was such a smart decision." Her sobbing continued. I waited until she calmed down before adding, "Mom, it will be okay, you can drive out to Winterhaven Manor and visit him every day, and not have to worry about the sleepless nights anymore."

"Well, I'll be bringing him home in ten days, anyway," she stated with authority, sobs now stifled.

Even though she made this statement, I believe on some level Mom knew that she wasn't going to leave him there just for "day care" or only one week, but that thought possibly made the transition easier for her. I wonder how she told him. I wonder what he said. She had made a difficult decision (or perhaps they had made it together?) and my hope was they'd both be safer now, and I'd no longer have to worry about the possibility of my dad falling and hurting either himself or her.

The ten days passed. Dad did not come home. Mom didn't say anything about bringing him home, and neither did I. My dad evidently did not mind the change. He had always been such an easy-going man, and with his memory loss, appeared to have no adjustment issues. Without verbalizing it, Mom also seemed to adjust to the change, and after a few days I think she began to enjoy her freedom.

Looking back, I can see that Mom had gradually become more afraid to leave Dad alone. He tended to forget he couldn't walk, and she feared he'd stand up, tip over, and she'd come home to find him on the ground injured—or worse.

49

She restricted her outings to absolutely necessary trips to the grocery store or to pick up the mail at their post office box. Now that Dad was in the nursing home, she could once again go to church on Sundays or to her friend's home for bridge games, and not feel anxious about Dad while she was away.

"Vicki, I am so busy, I almost forgot to go to the Manor and take the newspaper out to your Dad. I went to the grocery store this morning, and played bridge at Margaret's this afternoon. We were playing our last hand and I thought, good night, I didn't get the paper out to your dad!" She seemed at times almost buoyant when we spoke on the phone.

My mom had never lived on her own before, having married at 17, shortly after high school graduation in June of 1936. She grew up on a farm south of Nelson City, attending a one-room schoolhouse with her brother and several children from neighboring farms. After graduating from eighth grade, the only option for continuing her education was to go to the high school in town. A year prior, Bob, her only sibling, opted to quit school after completing the eighth grade, but she had bigger plans, and wanted to finish high school. There was no way for her to go back and forth from the farm to high school each day, so she lived with a family in Nelson City, offering babysitting services in exchange for room and board. On occasion, she caught a ride home to the farm for the weekend when she could find someone she knew who was going that way.

She met my father, who lived in Nelson City and was nearly six years her senior, sometime during her sophomore year in high school. It wasn't long before they were an "item." Mom often shared memories of her early infatuation by this most handsome and dashing older man. In my memory, Dad always treated Mom with respect and love, even when she was at her worst. I never remember him raising his voice to her, or anyone, for that matter, in anger.

Mom had aspirations for herself after high school graduation. She repeated the story to me many times over the years how she had desperately yearned to go to school to be a nurse, but when she shared this desire with her parents, they told her they didn't have the money for her to attend nursing school. The only option was for Mom to stay and help out on the farm. She was then adamant that she attend business school instead, as it cost less. "No," was her parents' firm reply, "You are needed on the farm." It was the middle of a depression, after all. She was 17 and ready for life, however, and her "life" did *not* include staying on the farm with her family. Mom's nurse practitioner related to me a story Mom had shared with her. "Harry wouldn't leave me alone. He pursued me, and pursued me, until I finally gave in and married him. At least it got me off the farm."

It was certainly not the best reason for getting married. Mom lived with regrets her entire life, and she had no compunction about sharing them with us over the years. Her regrets manifested in different ways, with verbal assaults most popular, directed towards Dad, my brother, or me. "You don't appreciate me." "*Your* Dad never appreciates anything I do for him!" "No one appreciates me!" "*Your* Dad never lifts a finger to help me. I never should have married him." "Someday I'm just going to walk out of here and never come back." My mother was an unhappy woman for most of her life, and it played out in her behavior towards others, but mostly in her behavior toward our family.

This interlude of diminished stress after Dad moved to the nursing home lasted less than two months.

"Vicki?"

"Hello, Mom, what's up?" It was almost the middle of October.

"The nursing home called just now to tell me your dad fell and broke his hip. He's in the hospital."

Whaaat? Wasn't he supposed to be **safer** *in the nursing home?* "Mom, what happened?"

"Well, they told me he tried to get up last night and walk to the bathroom by himself, and fell." The floors were institutional linoleum, not carpet. If he had been at home, it probably wouldn't have happened. I was suddenly overcome with regret for having been so insistent that Mom move Dad somewhere "safer."

"Oh, that's terrible news. I am so sorry."

The statistics for survival for a 91-year-old with a broken hip were not good, but my father, who was made of tough stuff, surprised us all, and steadily began to recover. Every day, Mom drove herself to visit him while he was in the hospital. She continued this pattern when he was moved back into the nursing home. As Dad recovered, he was able to walk short distances, but only with assistance. It became apparent that for all intents and purposes, he had become an invalid, confined to a wheelchair, except for brief moments on assisted, short walks. As always, he issued no verbal complaints over his unfortunate circumstances. He continued to enjoy meals, television, crossword puzzles, and visits from Mom.

As winter approached, I began making cautious overtures to Mom about moving them into an assisted-living facility in Coulson, thinking that maybe they could live together again, provided they had adequate assistance. I knew it would be a lot less stressful for all of us. My mother had other ideas. She was adamant about not leaving the area where she had spent her entire 86 years of life.

Around this time, I began receiving troubling reports from the staff at Winterhaven Manor.

"I'm calling to share our concerns regarding your mother. When she arrived at our facility today to visit your father, she looked as if she hadn't combed her hair, and she had on two mismatched earrings. Her clothes were wrinkled, and her appearance unkempt. Most of us who work here have known your mother a long time, and this seems so out of character for her. We're becoming concerned about her ability to properly care for herself."

This was troubling to me as Mom always took great pride in her appearance. Each week she made the trek to the local beauty shop, where her hairdresser teased and hair-sprayed her permed blonde hair into a bouffant coiffure. Mom loved nice clothes, jewelry, and trying any new gimmick to stay in shape that she might read about in one of her women's magazines. Her skin seemed to belie her years as it appeared smooth, with few wrinkles, perhaps from the myriad of lotions and potions she applied to her face on a daily basis.

The next day, I received another call. "Hi, I'm calling from the nursing home in Nelson City. I want to reassure you this call isn't about your dad, as he's doing very well. It's about your mother. We've been observing her driving, and it's become a major concern. When she leaves, we all hold our breaths watching her drive her car out of our parking lot, often screeching the tires, and driving off at a furious speed. We always say a prayer that she arrives home safely."

She had always been a "fast" driver (talking the local police officer out of speeding tickets was her specialty), but now I was hearing reports that she was sailing through intersections without slowing down, and generally terrorizing the streets. Lionel and I realized we were getting close to the dreaded, yet inevitable, intervention.

"Hi Mom. How are you doing today?"

"I'm okay. I just got back from visiting your Dad. Those girls! They don't know how to shave him right. I get so mad at them. They waste things too."

"What are you having for dinner?" I asked in an attempt to redirect the conversation away from her constant complaints about Dad's care.

"Oh, I have leftovers in the refrigerator."

"Like what?" I asked.

"I don't know, but don't worry honey, I could stand to lose some weight."

Mom was doing all her own housekeeping, grocery shopping, and cooking, and I don't think she was eating much or very well. This was later confirmed at a doctor's appointment when we learned she was at least ten pounds lighter than her normal weight.

"Uh, Mom, what would you think of you and Dad moving somewhere where you could be together?"

"I am NOT moving."

I am sure she found my suggestion annoying, but I found her stubbornness exasperating.

"Mom, I'm so worried about you being alone in the condo. I know everyone else who lives in the complex are gone for the winter. I also worry about you driving on icy roads to visit Dad."

"I'll be fine. You don't need to worry."

"Mom, promise me if the roads get too icy, you will think about moving, okay?"

Begrudgingly, she responded, "Okay."

I tried many different approaches to persuade her that it was a good idea to move closer to me. She would have none of it, and we reached a stalemate. I must admit at times I felt frustrated that she wouldn't listen to what I thought was common sense. Perspective has shed a completely different light on this time period for me, as I now have a better understanding of just how much the Alzheimer's affected her ability to reason.

Looking back on that time, I didn't truly grasp how amazing it was that she was able to hold things together for as long as she did. It's with a bit of awe that I realize how thankful I should be that something disastrous didn't happen. She might have had a car accident, killing herself or someone else, or she might have burned down their condo with the iron or stove left on.

"Hi Mom. I've been trying to call you for quite a while, and wondered where you were. It's dark outside!"

"Well, it snowed a few inches, and there wasn't anyone but me to shovel the sidewalk and driveway." This information really rattled me.

"Mom, surely there is some young person in your neighborhood or from church that we could hire to do the shoveling! I'm so worried that you might slip on the ice, and fall and break a bone. How about if I try and hire someone?"

"I've been doing this for a long time, and I am *not* going to fall and break something." She continued in a more subdued tone, "Besides, I really don't know of anyone around here that you could hire."

I'm sure I sounded like her parent, constantly worrying about her and her whereabouts. Within the group of condos in which my parents resided, she was the only one who didn't move south for the winter. Had she fallen, she could have lain there for hours before someone found her. To assuage my fears, I called every evening to be sure she was okay. I also called people I knew in Nelson City asking if they knew someone I could hire to shovel her walks, but I had no luck finding anyone. A feeling of helplessness washed over me as I imagined her slipping and falling into a snow bank, and either breaking her hip or freezing to death before anyone found her.

Once again, circumstances intervened. Winter weather continued with a vengeance. It was a bitterly cold, snowy winter with layers of ice on the streets, which my mother admitted scared her. Somehow, our earlier conversation must have had an impact, because out of nowhere she suddenly agreed to move.

EIGHT
Moving Quickly Before She Changes Her Mind

Crystal balls are only imaginary, but it sure would have been great to have had one when it came time to select an assisted-living facility! In retrospect, I didn't select the best facility for my parents' needs. At the time, however, it appeared to be the best option. I unwittingly chose the equivalent of a small, shiny, turquoise box with a white ribbon from the jewelry store, being sure it was from Tiffany's, only to open it and find a pair of knock-off generic earrings I didn't really like.

Mom and I talked over the possibilities. I was not in favor of them staying in Nelson City, although believe me, I have rethought this more than a few times since then. Today my heart tells me I made the right decision in moving them closer to me, but there were times throughout my mother's illness that I honestly wished she was still two hours away. That thought was a reflection of my own inability to cope with her behavior, and given their circumstances, it wouldn't have been practical to leave them in their hometown. In fairness, however, I did assess the facility in Nelson City, and learned what type of care was available for Mom. We visited Winterhaven Manor, and were shown a small, dark, and uninviting one-room apartment, a couple halls away from Dad. To me, it looked grim, and I simply could not envision my mother living in such a depressing environment. Living at Winterhaven Manor was as expensive as the facilities I had contacted in my hometown, which were newer, and certainly more inviting.

For the past year, between earning his undergraduate degree and entering medical school, my son Kyle worked as a caregiver at Cedar Grove, a newly opened assisted-living facility in our city. I remember visiting him at work, getting the "grand tour" of Cedar Grove and telling him, "If your Grandma and Grandpa ever have to move to an assisted-living facility, I would like it to be this one." It seemed no expense was spared in designing Cedar Grove; it was appealing and tastefully decorated, and didn't have that uneasy "institutional" feeling assisted-living facilities sometimes have.

Each hallway had an alcove, which was duly appointed a theme reflective of a different era, in keeping with what my parents' generation would best remember. There was a fishing nook, a sewing nook, a gardening nook, a birding nook, and a cowboy nook. Antiques abounded in the décor. The carpeted apartments were modern, light, and airy, and upon request included electric, freestanding fireplaces, each with a mantel, fake logs, and glass door. There were tiny kitchenettes, complete with microwave ovens and small refrigerators. Some apartments even had their own stackable washers and dryers. This seemed an appropriate living space for Mom, a place where she could maintain a sense of independence and self-respect.

Now that the time had come to select a facility for my parents, Cedar Grove seemed to be the logical choice. I decided to do some comparison "shopping," however, and toured several other facilities, meeting with their marketing representatives. Nothing I saw could come close to comparing with Cedar Grove. I called Cedar Grove and made an appointment to speak with their marketing director. She invited me to join her for lunch in the main dining room. I had heard from others that this facility had the best chef of all the assisted-living facilities in Coulson, so I was eager to sample their cuisine. I was not disappointed with the meal—it was delicious! I decided even I would like to live there!

But one important detail I forgot was that one should never judge a book by its cover. By the time my son Kyle had left Cedar Grove to attend medical school, this facility had moved through two administrators and a large number of staff members. At the time of his departure, Kyle had worked there for a year, and was one of the longest-employed caregivers in the building. My son is very even-keeled, and worked many double shifts when people didn't show up for work, or quit unexpectedly. I've heard that employee turnover is a chronic problem in many long-term care facilities. This kind of work appears to quickly weed out people who are not well -suited to it. It's a challenging job, to say the least. I think Kyle was able to continue with this job because he knew it was temporary, but maybe more importantly, because he developed loving relationships with several of the residents.

The issues associated with high employee turnover are an aspect of Cedar Grove that was not apparent on the surface. Even though I remembered Kyle working double shifts and hearing about all the people who quit over that year, I didn't realize what that instability might be like for the residents who lived there—especially those already suffering from dementia. A resident might bond with certain caregivers, only to see them disappear within a few weeks or months, replaced by new caregivers. This turnover could be very difficult for the residents, who thrived on familiarity and repetition.

These thoughts were the furthest thing from my mind during the luncheon that day with the marketing director.

"My parents will need an apartment on the assisted-living side so that Dad can get the extra care he will need. Will that be possible?"

"Yes, I'm sure it will. The only thing we'll need first is to have a nursing assessment from his current facility showing how much care he needs. It shouldn't be a problem."

I requested a two-bedroom apartment so that Mom wouldn't be awakened during the night when caregivers came in to assist my father in using the toilet. The marketing director showed me one of the available two-bedroom apartments, and as Goldilocks said, it looked "just right."

I also met with Mary James, the new administrator at Cedar Grove. We had an enjoyable visit and discovered we had much in common. "Since your son worked here, Vicki, we would like to offer your parents a monthly discount on their rent." I felt enthused and excited by the many activities, programs, and opportunities for Mom to get out and about and, of course, the food!

Over the course of several telephone conversations with Mom, I described Cedar Grove to her. "Mom, it's beautiful there. You and Dad can live together in the same apartment, each with your own bedroom. You can even have a fireplace! You'll be amazed at all the different activities there are at Cedar Grove. They even have a bus to take residents to appointments and shopping. There's also a group that plays bridge."

I think it was the bridge that sold her.

We started the application process. As I mentioned, the plan included my parents living in the same apartment, with daily assistance for my father. That would be the "assisted" living part of the plan, as Mom was still fairly independent. I paid the deposit to hold the apartment, and completed the assorted amalgamation of paperwork—the beginning of what would be a long paperwork trail I would navigate on their behalf over the years to come.

The next step involved the nursing assessment by the staff at Winterhaven Manor to determine the level of care necessary for Dad. The results brought about the first glitch in my plans.

It was the moment when I learned the shiny turquoise box with the white ribbon was not from Tiffany's after all.

Winterhaven Manor's report stated that my father needed too much skilled nursing care to be able to live with Mom on the assisted-living side of Cedar Grove. The only choice was for Mom to have her own apartment, and for Dad to live in "The Cottage," a nice and friendly name they had given the lock-down Alzheimer's unit.

The news was a disappointment, but by this time I had already been seduced by the possibilities Cedar Grove offered, and like a blinded lover moves forward in an unhealthy relationship, I moved forward with my parents' relocation to Cedar Grove. I expected explaining this turn of events to Mom would be a sad and tearful conversation, but she seemed to understand. In fact, she seemed relieved that she wouldn't be so responsible for Dad's care. In the few months he had lived in the nursing home, I believe she came to understand the toll it had taken on her mental and physical health. Still, in some ways, I felt like I had pulled a "bait and switch" number on Mom, because part of the enticement I had dangled before her to move to Coulson was that they could live together again. At least she could still play bridge …

It hindsight, it *was* the best choice to separate my parents because it quickly became apparent that my mother, even with assistance, could not be with my father 24/7. Actually, my mother's nurse practitioner had also said that my mother needed her own space where she didn't have to deal with my father and his disabilities 24 hours a day. I soon realized the wisdom of this statement. It would have made no sense to put Mom back in nearly the same detrimental situation she'd been in at their condo. The healthiest plan for her was to visit him, and then return to her own apartment. At least they would live in the same facility and she wouldn't be out terrorizing the town with her scary driving each day on her way to see him! Still …

Lessons Learned

When selecting an assisted-living or care facility, be aware of the specific care needs of your loved one(s) in order to best match them to the proper facility. Do not be seduced by outer trappings at assisted-living facilities. Fully investigate any facility by asking the facility, as well as yourself, important questions.

The Facility

- Is it located where you will be easily able to visit?

- Is it licensed? What are the regulatory agency ratings?

- Is there a memory-care unit available for people who are unable to live on their own?

- Is there a security system in place, especially in the evenings?

- Is there on-site care available, such as a visiting podiatrist? Is there a registered nurse on staff? Will you be responsible for your loved one taking medications or will the facility dispense them?

- What is the physical layout of the building and ease of movement between rooms and eating/recreation area?

Visit the facility at different times of the day and observe the residents and facility for cleanliness and general atmosphere.

The Care

- Ask for and follow-up on references.
- What is the turnover for residents and caregivers?
- Observe the attitudes of the caregivers; do you sense an attitude of empathy?
- What types of recreational activities are available for the residents?
- Does the facility have a bus available to take the residents out and about?
- Does the facility have a vehicle (i.e. special transport) that can assist residents in attending doctor's appointments?
- Eat a meal or two at the facility so you can see if the meals are well-balanced and acceptable.
- How often do monthly rates increase? Annually? Semi-annually? This helps your financial planning long-term.
- Are there any special requirements for medication acquisition and distribution? Are you allowed to bring in their medications, if so desired?
- What are the expectations, if any, for the family members? Should they stay out of the way, or can they be involved in the care of their loved one?
- Will your loved one be happier in a large facility with a lot of activity, or a smaller, more intimate setting that offers more calm and quietude?

NINE
Uprooted

We were soon faced with selling my parents' car and furniture, as well as sorting, packing, or giving away a lifetime of belongings. We also put their condominium up for sale.

Within a week of placing the ad Mom and I wrote in the Nelson City newspaper, I received a phone call. "Vicki, guess what? I just sold the car!" Mom sounded invigorated. "They're paying me almost full asking price. They'll even let me keep it until we move, so I can still go see Dad and take him the newspaper everyday. And, yesterday I sold the coffee tables to this sweet girl. She liked the crystal candy dish I had sitting on the one table, so I just gave her that too." The increased social contact was certainly having a positive effect on her mood.

More than once during this time, I felt the presence of guardian angels. I was bemused by the fact she was also giving extra belongings to whomever she sold items. This behavior was not in keeping with her depression-era personality of holding onto things, but ultimately it meant less to pack and move! Maybe there was still some element of logic in her way of thinking.

Plans were made for the move during the third weekend in January. The Sunday prior to the scheduled move, Lionel and I drove to Nelson City to help Mom with packing. It could not have been a worse weekend to be on the freeway. All along the two-hour trip, we prayed our car engine wouldn't freeze up—the temperature that winter day was 34 below zero. We were so relieved to turn off the freeway to Nelson City, but our safe arrival didn't diminish the funny lump of anxiety I felt in my stomach. I had no idea what to expect. Gingerly, we stepped up the icy staircase and entered the two-bedroom condo, immediately noticing Mom had done little in the way of packing. She had only partially packed three boxes with some random articles. In retrospect, I'm sure this lack of packing demonstrated that she was undoubtedly frustrated and confused by the process, but her acting skills were quite polished, so she displayed neither of those emotions that day. I had definitely not made the adjustment in my thinking that my mother's organizational skills were on the decline, and I was actually a bit puzzled and, although I didn't show it, almost irritated that she had done so little to get ready.

"Vicki, I want you to take whatever you want," Mom was quick to say, as Lionel and I put together the first box of the day with some strong tape. I looked around me and felt suddenly sad. My mom was disassembling her life, one box at a time. Looking up, I saw a familiar ceramic hummingbird figurine sitting on the fireplace in the living room. "Oh Mom, do you remember when I gave you that hummingbird?" I asked her, my eyes becoming moist. She looked at me blankly, obviously having no idea, but I remembered exactly when I had given it to her on Mother's Day many years ago. My first daughter was only one month old, and Mom and Dad had come to visit. The hummingbird was the first memento of the day I lovingly wrapped in packing paper and placed into my own box of treasures.

As with most people who have lived in one place for many years, my parents had collected and saved a myriad of odd possessions, some of which I didn't even recognize. There was nothing to do but dig in and start sorting. Mom became our "sidewalk supervisor" for the afternoon.

"Um, Mom, do you want these?" I asked her, holding up two partially full cardboard boxes of poker chips. She laughed and said, "No, I don't think I'll be needing those." For some reason, I couldn't put both boxes of poker chips in the discard pile and although I'm not a poker player, found myself putting one of the cardboard boxes in "my" box because of my memories of Dad teaching his three small grandchildren how to play "21" so many years ago.

When I moved into the kitchen to begin emptying drawers and cupboards, I opened the drawer where Mom had always kept her paperwork, such as bills and receipts. I was astonished to see the disarray, and wondered how she managed to pay her bills on time. Calling it "a little disorganized" was a gross understatement. I sorted as I went, and hoped I didn't find a stack of unpaid, overdue bills.

As we sorted, wrapped, and packed that afternoon, Mom brought up a subject that had become uncomfortably familiar to me. Over the previous few weeks, she had started making negative statements about my brother's lack of involvement, and as the moving day had grown closer, she had become brazenly angry with him because he had not made plans to come home to help with the move. She was adamant. "Now, Vicki, I want you to take all of our money that's left when we die. I don't want that damn brother of yours to have anything. He didn't even show up to help with this moving mess."

"Mom," I reassured her for the umpteenth time, "we'll probably spend it all on living expenses for you and Dad. You won't have to even worry about this, okay?" I then attempted to change the subject. Little did I know, this conversation would repeat itself obsessively over the next two years. She was almost always rude to my brother when he called, and often would hang up on him, or say cruel things. I'm certain this behavior was more related to her dementia than anything else. Something else I did not yet know was that ultimately, I would become the object of her anger, and my brother would suddenly—and inexplicably—regain her good graces.

One of the more daunting tasks that cold winter's day was cleaning out their enormous storage area on the main level of the complex. My parents' condo was adjacent to the town's golf course, so Dad stored his golf cart in this large room. The storage area held almost as many memories for me as their living space. Growing up, my three children considered this storage room a magical place to play, where they discovered new treasures in the numerous boxes, the old footlocker, and an antique dresser stored there. Treasures that sparked their imagination included cast-off clothing, crocheted dolls, antique books, golf balls and tees in several empty Folgers coffee cans, an assortment of old tools, and outdated house wares.

I opened the footlocker. "Oh Mom, what shall we do with all these old *Life* magazines? Wow! Here's one from JFK's assassination. Oh, and look at this one! It talks about the opening of Disneyland!" Some of the magazines were 50 or more years old.

"Well, like I said before, Vicki, if you want 'em, take 'em." Into my box went the Life magazines.

"I love this old chest of drawers. I wish I had somewhere to put it in my house," I sighed as I began to clean out the rickety drawers, knowing the chest was destined for the charity pile.

Mom helped us to the best of her ability, and appeared to handle the chaos in a business-like, detached manner. By the time Lionel and I had to leave that day, we felt we'd accomplished quite a lot. Whatever was left could be easily packed after we arrived on Saturday morning of the following weekend. Looking at the mountain of boxes in her living room as we put on our coats, Lionel and I turned to each other with the question, "How do two people accumulate so much … stuff?!"

Thankfully, the next weekend's weather was a total opposite extreme of 60 degrees—one can never predict weather in our state in January, but this was unseasonably warm. No ice or snow greeted us that day as we walked up the condo steps. Mom was waiting, and seemed excited to embark on the day's new adventure. "I've been so busy this week!" she announced as we walked through the door. "They picked up the car yesterday afternoon, and I gave them a couple of old, wool blankets. You never know when you might get stuck on the road in bad weather and need to keep warm." Mom always tried to be helpful. "I packed a couple more boxes too, mostly odds and ends from the hall closet to get rid of. What a bunch of junk in there!"

A friend from Coulson had loaned us his Suburban with a trailer hitch. Lionel backed our rented U-Haul as close as possible to the condo's back door. We had already marked the boxes for donation, and Mom watched dispassionately as we filled the 16-foot trailer with those boxes, furniture and other miscellaneous, no-longer-needed items. Much to my relief, partway through this operation, my cousin and some friends from Nelson City arrived to help us. It was mid-afternoon when, Lionel, Mom, and I pulled away from the condo to make a rather large delivery to the local Goodwill. The store volunteers helped us unload box after box, along with the furniture, into their warehouse. By now all three of us were so tired that I'm not sure we even registered the magnitude of what was really happening. My parents' home had been dismantled forever. I found myself repeating, *it's only stuff … it's only stuff … and with the move, I'll be able to take better care of them.* Mom showed no reaction.

With that mission completed, the three of us drove back to the condo. Lionel and I loaded all the remaining boxes and most of the remaining furniture into the newly emptied U-Haul.

Our next project was cleaning. While I combed both the condo and storage area looking for any missed minutia, Lionel vacuumed, filled nail holes, and took out trash. We scrubbed cupboards, cleaned toilets, tub, and shower, wiped down walls, counter-tops, and closet shelves, hoping our attention to detail might hasten a buyer.

As nightfall descended on this most exhausting day, Lionel and I took my mother to dinner. We sank into the restaurant chairs, and discussed our successful day. "How're you feeling, Mom?" I asked her, as she hadn't said much all day. "Oh, mostly I'm tired to the bone, honey. Let's just eat, go home and go to bed, okay? I'm beat." That was fine with me! I can't even remember what we ate. I do remember all three of us collapsed into our beds as soon as we arrived back at the condo. I fell into a deep, uninterrupted slumber, the type of sleep that only exhaustion creates. It was a much bigger project than we had envisioned. Talking about moving, and then physically doing it in a weekend, are two completely different things.

Awakening groggily from our slumber early the next morning, we finished packing the rest of the furniture into the U-Haul, including Mom's bed frame and mattress and the pullout sofa where we had been sleeping only a couple of hours earlier. We ate a relatively silent breakfast, each seemingly lost in our own thoughts. When Lionel, Mom, and I walked out the door of the condo for the last time, Mom didn't look back. I did. There were a lot of memories, both happy and sad, made there in the past 27 years.

We had one last stop as we left town, and that was to gather up my dad and his few belongings at Winterhaven Manor.

"Hi Dad. How'd you like to take a drive?" He was sitting in his wheelchair in the common area of the Manor taking a nap, chin on chest, a shock of his thick white hair falling lazily over one of his bushy eyebrows. *What a handsome man he still is,* I thought as I walked over, leaned down, and gave him a kiss.

He looked up at me and smiled. We gathered up the small collection of possessions waiting in his room, signed the appropriate discharge forms, and loaded it all into the Suburban.

The two-hour drive from Nelson City to Coulson was actually quite restful, but we didn't have time to be tired, or enjoy our rest, because our job was only partially complete. Upon arrival in Coulson came the unloading, unpacking, and settling of Mom and Dad into their new "home." Thank goodness for our wonderful friends who met us at the facility and showered blessings upon us with their help. Since Mom and Dad would be located in different areas of the building, his belongings went one way to "The Cottage" and hers the opposite way, to her third-floor, corner, one-bedroom apartment.

Upon arrival in The Cottage, I immediately was stricken with an unsettling premonition that perhaps the Alzheimer's unit was not the best place for Dad. Even though he did have the dementia component of Parkinson's disease, he was definitely not an "escape" risk, as many of the other residents proved to be. Most of the people in this part of the facility had fairly severe Alzheimer's disease. Many of them were completely demented and acted out in very strange ways, much like mischievous toddlers. There were, however, other residents in this area who seemed similar to Dad's level of functioning, so I hoped he might interact with them, although most of them were women. His dementia at this time was very mild—mostly confusion, which would certainly be normal for any elderly person who had been moved twice within a few months.

After arranging Dad's belongings in his room, Mom and I sat with him in the central gathering area of The Cottage for a while. We wanted to be sure he felt comfortable before Mom went back to her apartment and I went home for the evening. Another gentleman was sitting amongst the residents, and we had a nice conversation.

"Hello, where do you all come from?"

"Oh, we're from Nelson City," said Mom.

"Really? Well, I know some people from Nelson City," and he went on to name several. We visited for a few minutes, and Mom and I relaxed. I attempted to console myself that The Cottage was filled with possibilities. After all, kind people like this gentleman visited residents here and carried on interesting conversations. It wasn't until a couple of days later that we learned this nice gentleman, dressed so meticulously in a checkered shirt, V-necked sweater, pressed slacks and dress shoes, was actually a Cottage resident, and not a visitor at all! Sometimes it is not apparent whose dementia is severe enough to warrant living in a "Cottage-level" care unit.

The Cottage layout was conveniently arranged, with a large and comfortable gathering area filled with plush recliners and couches, and bordered by a communal dining area. There was also an area off to one side decorated like a living room where residents gathered to watch TV. The individual rooms were in pods of two or three, each grouped along the outside wall in a large square, with the common areas serving as an indoor courtyard of sorts. Like the rest of Cedar Grove, each hallway in The Cottage was replete with a thematic alcove.

Unlike the rest of the facility's alcoves, however, those in The Cottage more closely resembled children's play areas than areas designed to "comfort" an aging generation. There was a nook with a "workbench" filled with plastic hammers, wrenches, screwdrivers, and other assorted plastic tools for the residents' use. Another hallway had dolls and doll cribs, a plastic iron, ironing board, and washtub. There was a hallway adorned with hats, shawls, and other dress-up clothing items. My dad's favorite nook became the one filled with stuffed animals. Like a small child, he later adopted one of the stuffed dogs, which he usually carried cradled in his arms or sitting atop his lap. On any given day, the dog had a different name, ranging from Fido to Elwood. The tactile stimulation provided by the stuffed animals certainly seemed to touch a chord in my dad. He loved his stuffed dog.

Lessons Learned

if you need help, ask for it! Moving is stressful under any circumstances, but more so when you are moving someone from a home they have occupied for many years into a small apartment or a single room. It would have been helpful if we had had more days to prepare for and execute the move. When preparing for a move, assess how much space will be available in the new living space and sort possessions into groups: move, donate, or trash. For the larger or more valuable items being left behind, a "sell" group is advisable. This very possibly will include a car. Be wary of bringing jewelry or other valuables to the facility, as many possessions can go missing in an assisted-living facility where residents suffer from some form of dementia. Perhaps suggest to your loved one that you purchase a small safe or that you keep the items for them at your residence.

TEN
The Reality of Moving

Oh, the dreams I had, with my parents now living in the same city as me for the first time in 35 years. I envisioned Mom in my kitchen baking her famous chocolate chip cookies; I could practically smell the wonderful aroma of these freshly baked cookies wafting through my house. How idyllic it would be! I fantasized about her and Dad sitting at our dining room table for dinners that we would prepare together, or them spending an afternoon now and then at my home. Somehow I had not taken into account that my house was inaccessible for a wheelchair … my blissful reverie was shattered as I quickly began to recognize my misconception of reality.

I still saw my mother as basically "normal," with some forgetfulness. Reality was that whenever I invited Mom to my house she never acted interested. "Oh Vicki, you live too far from here to come all the way over to get me and then have to bring me back. Besides, your dad might need something, and what would he do if I wasn't here?" *(It was only five miles to my house, so this reaction was possibly the result of having lived in a small town all her life.)*

"Mom, of course it isn't too far! I would love to come get you and bring you over here for a few hours. If Dad needs something, he is surrounded by helpers."

The few times she *did* come, she complained, "Vicki, your house is just too damn cold for me," even though she was sitting by the warmth of the gas fireplace or a space heater, or "I think it's probably time for me to get home," acting anxious. We tried shopping outings instead, which she obviously enjoyed, but this became difficult as her mobility steadily declined. Thank goodness for electric carts some stores have available, as these outings would have been impossible without them. She loved maneuvering the cart through the store, and only occasionally ran into things.

Because of Dad's wheelchair, it wasn't possible to bring him to my house unless someone could carry him up our stairs. The choices were either twelve stairs up to my front sidewalk or a narrow stairway coming into the kitchen from the back door. Neither was suited to a handicapped person in a wheelchair. Aside from this blatantly obvious problem, he also became agitated within 30 minutes of arriving, asking to "go home." Why had I thought it would be different when they lived here? Like stars at daybreak, one by one, I slowly began to let my dreams and expectations fade away.

Lessons Learned

Release any expectations of what you imagine life will be like once your loved one moves into an assisted-living or care facility. Expectations do nothing but cause unrealistic hopes and heartbreak. Learn to go with the flow—this took me a long time!

ELEVEN
Doctor Visits

After they had settled into their new home, the seemingly endless rounds of doctor visits began. My parents had always been in good physical health, but over the course of the last several years had neglected certain aspects of preventive health. I decided to improve their lives, with the intention of remedying any existing neglect. I thought good physical health might help improve their quality of life, allowing them to be with me longer. The realization that was slow in coming was no matter how sound their physical health remained, there was little I could do to prolong their mental acuity. I wasn't cognizant that they were moving to that plane of existence that only those with dementia can travel.

It was stressful for all three of us to visit the many specialty doctors. My parents hadn't been to a dentist in years. My father's new dentist told us, "Mr. Andersen, you have nine cavities. You also have five teeth diseased beyond repair, which, unfortunately, need to be pulled. I'm sorry to tell you that includes one of your front teeth." Dad smiled, seemingly oblivious to the implications of this news. The whole process involved several trips to the oral surgeon, and additional unwanted stress. Mom's teeth were in better condition, but she also needed several teeth pulled, meaning even more trips to the oral surgeon.

Usually, I drove and helped my parents to each doctor visit, but because of scheduling difficulties for one of the visits to the oral surgeon, the Cedar Grove van dropped them off while I was at work at the pediatric clinic helping moms and babies learn to breastfeed. I had been somewhat nervous about this situation, wondering if they would successfully get in and out of the office on their own. The Cedar Grove bus driver assured me she would walk in with my parents and help them get registered, and then return to the office to retrieve them when they were finished. What could go wrong?

Apparently, everything could go wrong.

The day of their appointment I received a call at work from the oral surgeon's office, "Hi, I'm calling from Dr. Richland's office." Immediately, I developed an uneasy feeling in the pit of my stomach.

The receptionist went on to say, "We just sent your parents back to Cedar Grove in the van."

"Yes?"

"We weren't able to do any dental work on your father."

"You weren't? Why not?" I imagined that he had fallen ill or something.

"Well, your mother wouldn't let us come near him. She was adamant that he did not need any dental work done."

Astonished, I replied, "Oh no, really?" If only Mom had stayed behind at Cedar Grove! I knew, however, that she would never agree to remain behind while Dad went to an appointment. This incident was one of many that gave me a faint glimmer of how much the dementia was affecting her cognitive processes.

My dad's eye doctor visit was also disappointing. He confirmed an earlier doctor's diagnosis. "Your father has macular degeneration, and it's causing a gradual decline of his vision," explained the doctor.

"What can we do about it?" asked Mom.

"Well, unfortunately, there's no available treatment," and he then gently explained that my dad was going blind.

The orthopedic surgeon's visit was more positive.

"Well, Mr. Andersen, your hip is healing well. How'd you like to begin some physical therapy?"

My dad gave a positive response with a nod of his head.

The doctor directed his next comment to me. "Let's have the caregivers at Cedar Grove work with him, starting slow, by helping him walk around The Cottage using a walker."

That sounded great. Maybe he might actually start to move around on his own with a walker. We left this appointment with an air of encouragement.

Sadly, the walking "rehab" was not as successful as we'd hoped. Over time, it didn't amount to much more than standing, turning, and transferring with assistance. His days of walking on his own were indeed over. My father, however, never ceased talking about standing up and walking. "Help me up, will you?" were often the first words I heard when visiting him. I would patiently explain why that wasn't a good idea. After I finished my explanation, he usually looked me in the eye and asked, "Help me up, will you?"

Walking became an obsession for him, and because of the dementia, he never really seemed to understand that he could no longer walk on his own.

The results of our visit to the internal medicine doctor were also positive. He marveled at both my parents' good internal health, with normal blood pressure, heart rate, and blood work.

The results of Mom's visit to the arthritis doctor weren't as encouraging.

"Mrs. Andersen, we have the results of the Dexa-scan, and it shows a low bone density. You have osteoporosis. I recommend you begin taking a medication once a week that will help increase bone density while at the same time strengthen your bones, and hopefully decrease the possibility of bone fractures."

Well, that sounded good on paper, as they say. Reality was a completely different story. Our plan to help her remember to take the medication involved marking her calendar with a big star on the same day every week. We looked at the calendar together as I asked, "See the big black star on every Tuesday?" She nodded affirmatively. "You take this pill on Tuesday, the day that has a star on your calendar." She continued to nod. This plan worked erratically, at best. If I could have personally handed her the pill each week when I visited, it might have been successful. Unfortunately, she had to take the pill an hour before eating breakfast in the morning, and I was unable to be there at that time of day. Leaving her in charge of administering her own weekly medication, I learned, is an example of an unrealistic plan for someone with Alzheimer's disease.

Mom's arthritis caused persistent pain in her knees, fingers, neck, and shoulders. At her visit to an orthopedic surgeon, we heard, "Mrs. Andersen, unfortunately, if you look at this x-ray picture with me, you can see, just here," pointing to the film, "there's no cartilage left in your knee and you have bone rubbing against bone with every agonizing step. It is no wonder that it's painful! Short of a knee replacement, about the only other thing we can do is prescribe some pain medication." Sadly, the prescribed pain medication gave only limited relief.

Unfortunately, Mom's apartment at Cedar Grove was in the furthest corner from Dad's unit, and it was a long walk for her to reach his room. Because of the arthritis in her knee, it wasn't long before she started using a walker—another example of something she said she would *never* do. Her knee continued to splay out at an awkward angle, and her gait was reduced to a limp. Even with the pain medication, some degree of discomfort remained her constant companion.

Nevertheless, she persevered on her journey to The Cottage to visit Dad once or twice each and every day.

Lessons Learned

When arranging for doctor appointments for your loved one, be realistic and reevaluate your goals in making these visits. It wasn't until much later that I realized my parents weren't interested in going to all these appointments; they did it to please me.

If it will lower your stress level, by all means look into the possibility of someone other than your loved one administering their own medications in order to be certain the right dosages are given at the appropriate times. Although it was an attempt on my part to be frugal with their money (because this service is often an extra monthly charge in an assisted-living facility), in hindsight, it would have been the better choice.

TWELVE
Adjustments

There were many adjustments associated with my parents' move to Cedar Grove. Moving them away from all they had known for an entire lifetime was undoubtedly traumatic. I have no idea what my dad thought about the move. When I asked him questions, he only stared at me. Mom verbalized how much she missed her church family and her home. She didn't integrate with the other residents at the facility as I had hoped. She actually got into a fight with another resident who lived across the hall from her.

Mom's next-door neighbor, Darlene, was a very sweet, wrinkly, elderly lady who was deaf and had trouble walking, but wow, could she play the piano! Prior to my mother's arrival, Monica, the neighbor across the hall, typically brought Darlene the newspaper each day, and helped her to the dining room for mealtime. Monica had lived at the facility since it opened two years before, and was a fairly high-functioning elderly woman (translation: I could have a reasonable conversation with her), who still drove her own car, and lived at Cedar Grove for the social interaction. Mom and Monica were friendly, but Mom, the nurse wannabe, saw in the deaf Darlene someone she could take care of and began weaseling in on Monica's "territory."

"Well, Vicki, what a day I've had!" Mom exclaimed during our daily phone conversation. "I was downstairs in the sitting room, as usual, reading the newspaper, and when I finished, I remembered how much Darlene enjoys the paper, so thought I'd take it up to her." It had become something of a power struggle between Mom and Monica to see who brought Darlene the daily newspaper first, or who showed up at Darlene's door first to escort her to mealtime. "When I knocked on her door, wouldn't you know it, she already had a copy from Monica. I told Darlene I'd come back to get her for the noon meal. When I came back just before dinner, Monica was already knocking on her door, and when I said that I was going to help Darlene, Monica got mad at me! Vicki, we got in a fight!"

Evidently, they actually engaged in a shoving match over who was going to escort Darlene to the noon meal. "I finally backed off," Mom continued, "thinking if it's that important to her, she can just take Darlene. In fact, I'm done with the whole shootin' match. You aren't going to find me bringing newspapers, or even talking to either of them again." Mom was good at carrying a grudge. Eventually, however, all three seemed to forget that the altercation had even happened, and were friends again. Perhaps, at times, poor memories can actually be small blessings in disguise.

According to Henry Brodaty, professor of psychogeriatrics at the University of New South Wales, the more a person uses his or her brain doing activities, such as Sudoku, crosswords, playing bridge, or even learning a new language, the stronger the neural connections in the brain are likely to become. Even though my dad did several crossword puzzles every day, I haven't dwelt on the fact it didn't seem to help him—I've chosen to focus instead on Brodaty's information, so I am learning Spanish (*yo estoy aprendiendo Español*) to help keep *my* brain active.

Mom had enjoyed playing bridge for as long as I can remember, and simultaneously belonged to two or three clubs for many years. When I conducted my original facility search, several other assisted living facilities were immediately ruled out because there were no residents that played bridge. I knew how much Mom loved to play bridge, and how beneficial it was for her brain, so a huge selling point for Cedar Grove was the bridge players.

I remember Mom's excitement during my early visits. "Vicki, I have to show you something!" Mom exclaimed. She took my hand and led me into her bedroom where she opened her dresser drawer and pointed. There was an impressive pile of quarters she'd won playing bridge. It pleased me there was an activity at the facility in which she enjoyed participating. Unhappily, bridge was the next dream that evaporated. Within a few months of her arrival, one player's failing eyesight precluded her from participating, so the group was left one person short. Those remaining somehow figured out how to play with three people, although Mom confided that it "didn't work too well." I can only imagine what those card games were like! It wasn't long before one of the other regulars moved to The Cottage because of her advanced dementia. It appeared mom's card-playing days were over.

Another activity I encouraged Mom to become involved in was the Red Hat Society at Cedar Grove, part of a worldwide social organization for women over 50. The Red Hat Society is a group of women who embrace life by wearing purple dresses and red hats, who meet regularly to share lunch, laughs, and friendship. Even with much encouragement, and many invitations on the part of other women at the facility, Mom simply wasn't interested in joining this group.

In the beginning, she often played bingo at Cedar Grove, participated in some of the crafts, and attended the seated exercise classes several times a week. This seemed a good way for her to spend time out of her apartment and participate in something other than mealtime or sitting with Dad. Unfortunately, over time the pain in her knee bothered her too much to participate in the exercise classes and she lost interest in the crafts and bingo. Apparently, she was withdrawing into herself, and no encouragement from me made much difference. I mourned her withdrawal and spent fruitless nights waking around 2 or 3 a.m., wracking my brain to think of ways to help make her days more interesting. I seemed to have taken it upon myself to be the "provider" of entertainment options. I failed miserably at my job. This did *not* help the guilty conscience I continued to hone, nor did it help my tendency to second guess decisions regarding my parents' care. I was always asking myself if I'd made the right choices, or whether I was doing enough to help engage them in life.

When the Cedar Grove bus took residents to different stores every week, Mom often went along, and told me she enjoyed the outing, especially the "Only One Dollar" store. The time arrived, however, that even this enjoyment faded away, and she became more and more obsessive about spending the entire day in The Cottage sitting beside my dad.

Lessons Learned

no matter how much we hope to ease the transition for our loved ones, there is only so much that we can personally do. Realize that you are not the entertainment committee, and do not berate yourself that you are unable to be with your loved one 24/7.

THIRTEEN
The Colorful Cottage

There was definitely a range of dementia-affected people living in The Cottage. There were several people who appeared to be quite "normal," much like the gentleman we had met on our first evening in The Cottage. In particular, two ladies and one man in the cast of Cottage characters stand out in my mind. Ethel and Dolores, both teachers in their former lives, usually carried their purses everywhere, and were always tastefully dressed, as if ready to welcome their students on the first day of school. They were often found sitting together talking in the common area of The Cottage when I arrived to visit my dad. As they brought their heads close together in a conspiratorial manner to whisper unheard secrets, it reminded me of two teenage girls in a high school cafeteria.

Ethel and Dolores were able to come and go from The Cottage on the honor system to attend events in the main gathering room of the assisted living side of the building. Because they always returned on time, they were not considered flight risks. As a visitor to The Cottage, it was hard for me to imagine why they were there. Then there was Al, a plumber by trade, who for some unknown reason seemed to remember me each week. Al was friendly and liked to chat. He often sat in the TV room in "his" recliner writing in a journal or watching television. He could become unreasonably upset if someone else sat in his self-proclaimed chair, so people learned not to sit in that particular recliner if he was nearby. Ethel, Dolores, and Al were some of the more functional Alzheimer's patients in The Cottage.

There were also people living in The Cottage at the opposite end of the spectrum, oftentimes frighteningly so. Charles, a man living in the same pod as Dad, was extremely angry, and spent most of his time cursing and threatening people. Charles sometimes came into Dad's room and frightened Mom when she was there visiting, cursing and muttering to himself. Dwight, another resident, used a cane to walk, and sometimes, unprovoked, would start to wave it around frantically; it was important to move out of his way, as he paid no attention to those around him. Fortunately, in my experience, he always missed striking someone on the head, although often by a narrow margin. Elizabeth, a more severely disturbed resident, walked back and forth incessantly, her body bent almost in half, picking at her own clothing as well as others', mumbling incoherently. For the novice visitor, it was disconcerting to see her approach, especially when she reached out to pick some unseen piece of lint, or whatever it was only she could see, off the visitor's clothing. It was obvious that she was making conversation, but impossible to understand what she was saying or even to whom she was speaking. Bernice, with her red-rimmed and vacant eyes, liked to stand as close as possible to people, perhaps in an attempt to make a connection from her otherworldly existence. She never spoke, but looked pleadingly with such melancholy eyes, imploring us to unlock her silence.

Helen, on the other hand, rarely stopped talking with her sharp, scolding voice. I thought perhaps her outbursts were a subconscious manifestation of anguish over the state of her self-destructing brain. Her angry sentences started out with several coherent words, but then quickly lapsed into gibberish. One afternoon when we were in The Cottage visiting Dad, she came to stand beside us. One of her eyes was droopy and no longer opened, and the other fiery eye was trained on Dad, boring holes right through him. Her short, grey hair stood up in awkward angles all over her head, and she was wearing a pink sweatshirt, blue pants, and bright pink crocs.

"It's time to go home uleas picts simplet depolsy liptik!" she scolded Dad. Seemingly undisturbed, he tacitly nodded agreement. She grabbed his arm to pull him up, as Mom and I stared in disbelief.

As Helen tugged on his arms he began to stand up, even though he was unable to stand without support, let alone walk.

In a voice that was almost a shout, I blurted out, "Dad! Remember, you can't walk!"

"Oh," he exclaimed to Helen, "I can't walk!"

She looked at him with suspicion, and let him sit back into his chair. She then turned her attention to me.

"Well, aren't you just skurpy! You don't masu litper shit-nu, you witlin skurpy bilt," she spoke sharply to me, with her eyes piercing mine.

I wasn't sure what "skurpy" meant, but it was obvious it was not a compliment.

Looking back at Dad, she firmly stated, "We *need* to go home *now*! Let's go!"

Helen turned Dad's wheelchair around, as Mom and I watched with concern.

"Ouch! You are rolling over my toes!" Helen cried as Dad's wheelchair came into contact with her crocs.

Mom and I watched to see what would happen next. Helen managed to turn Dad's chair around, and he grabbed her arm as they moved to the other side of the room. Soon she lost interest in Dad, and he rolled away from her around the corner into the hallway. I started to get up to go and retrieve him, but one of the caregivers walked by, and wheeled him back to where Mom and I sat on the couch.

"Where did you disappear to?" I joked with him.

"I think he was hiding from Helen," offered the caregiver.

Jim, a retired engineer, was wheelchair-bound like my dad, but much more rambunctious. Whenever we saw Jim headed our way, we were careful to move aside as he was quite mobile and did not necessarily watch where he was going. Jim liked to talk, and was quite social, but asked the same questions repeatedly, so a visitor's social interaction depended on their range of patience for repetition. I saw that The Cottage maintenance people frequently repainted doorframes, walls, and wall trim. Jim was not alone in his contributions to these nicks and gashes in the facility, however, as I often also saw my dad bang into doorframes and walls with his wheel or footrest of his wheelchair.

When my mother and I visited Dad in The Cottage, the three of us generally sat at the dining room table for a snack together. Other residents would often join us at our table. Jim was a tablemate with Dad, so he often wheeled over and sat with us. He liked to play with the silverware, salt, pepper, and sugar packets, centerpiece, or any object inadvertently left on the table. It felt like there was a toddler in our midst. Mom found this understandably upsetting and often commented to me, "Your Dad does not belong with these people." I have to admit that over time I came to agree with her assessment, as it did remind me of Ken Kesey's book, *One Flew Over the Cuckoo's Nest*. It now occurred to me that my choice of a facility had not been in his best interests, even though he never said anything negative. Mom more than made up for his lack of communication regarding his living arrangements with her non-stop complaints, however. I sometimes thought back to when we made the original plans for my parents' move to Cedar Grove, and how my attempts to keep them together in the same apartment had failed when it became apparent the amount of skilled nursing care Dad required would necessitate him living in the Alzheimer's wing. Even though I had sensed somewhere in the back of my mind he might not really belong in The Cottage, the wheels were in motion, and I had simply accepted that is where he needed to live. For a long time, I was at a loss in thinking how I might change the situation for my dad. Moving them to a different facility was already a faint idea dancing in the back of my brain, but hadn't yet invaded my daily thoughts.

Lessons Learned

The cliché is true: you can't judge a book by its cover.

When considering a live-in care facility, remember how important it is to consider the social needs of your loved one, as well as his/her medical and physical needs.

If possible, take the time to visit the facilities you are considering for your loved one multiple times in order to observe the residents as well as the caregivers. This is something I neglected to do, resulting in Dad's "incarceration" with people in a much different mental state.

FOURTEEN
Save or Spend

Assisted living is NOT inexpensive. My parents were very fortunate to have amassed a quarter of a million dollars in their savings and investments over the years. They seldom traveled, and when they did it was usually to see my family or my brother's family. They also lived frugally. My encouragement to them over the years was consistent: "Travel, spend your money, enjoy life!" They did not listen to me. Now, in a twisted sense, their frugality became my salvation, and I'm *glad* they ignored my advice. Their financial prudence placed them in a secure financial position so they could afford a high-quality assisted-living facility rather than be forced to move in with me. I believe the consequence of this outcome saved my sanity. I realize many people do not have this luxury and I've read countless hair-raising tales of 24/7 caretaking for a relative with dementia. I continue to feel a tremendous sense of gratitude for my parent's thriftiness. Even though my parents rarely traveled, my mother suddenly began "remembering" that she and Dad traveled the world. She shared with me how glad she was that she and Dad went "everywhere" and saw "everything." I don't know where these memories came from, but I'm pleased she was able to reframe them to suit her and had no regrets for that part of her life. I believe these memories, fabricated as they may be, were a gift for her.

My parents did not intend on using their life savings for assisted living (I'm sure no one does). That possibility never arose in our conversations as they aged, because they were insistent they would "never move to a nursing home." I assume they planned to pass away tucked in the comfort of their own bed, in their own home, in their own town. On paper, they had carefully divided all their assets equally between my brother and me. Their plan was to bequeath an inheritance for their children, grandchildren, and great-grandchildren.

Reflecting on the reality of *my* parents' situation, thoughts of my future continue to haunt me. Have Lionel and I saved enough money? Are we living life to the fullest? There is a part of me that feels an indescribable panic and desire to "race the clock" and travel, spend money, and enjoy life while I am of "sound" mind. I find I am developing a devil-may-care attitude about saving a lot of money. On the other side of the coin, however, I also realize that I would never want to burden my children with 24/7 care-taking because I had not planned well. The solution for now has been to purchase long-term care insurance for Lionel and me, in addition to our IRAs. We're still planning and taking trips.

Lessons Learned

For peace of mind regarding your own future, this may be a good time to take stock of your finances, both present and future, and consider the possibility of long-term care insurance. Although it may not be a particularly comfortable conversation, if you have children, take the time to sit down with them and discuss your wishes for care in the event they might someday be your caregiver.

It is also a good time to recognize and remind yourself that *the life you are now living is not a dress rehearsal,* and try to reorient yourself to living, fully present in "the now."

FIFTEEN
Settling into the Routine

In the beginning, my visits to Cedar Grove occurred several times a week, but over time evolved to one afternoon a week. I was usually home from the office around lunchtime and Mom had no trouble remembering to call me after her noon meal on Thursdays, so I would leave my house soon after she phoned. While I was on my way, she washed her hair so by the time I arrived she was ready for me to transform myself into her amateur beautician. I rolled up her hair in old-fashioned curlers, dried it with a handheld hairdryer, and then styled it. I am certainly no beautician, and although she could have gotten a better "do" at the facility's in-house salon, she said she "didn't like the hairdresser" (of Hispanic heritage). I am sure that the reasons were much more related to money and racism than generalized dislike; she didn't like the thought of spending $14 for a shampoo and set, or having someone other than a Caucasian touch her hair. Rather than argue or cajole, it was easier for me to simply relent and be her hair stylist each week.

One afternoon as I was finishing my lunch, I heard the telephone ringing.

"Hello?"

"Well, I'm ready."

"Oh, hi, Mom. I'll head over to your house in just a few minutes. I'm almost done eating lunch. If you want to wait until I get there, I'll wash your hair for you today."

"No, I can do it."

"All right. I'll be there in 15 minutes."

Arriving at Cedar Grove, I parked in the front parking lot as always and dashed up the three flights of stairs to her apartment. There was an elevator, but I liked the stairs. As usual, she had left her front door ajar for me. Upon entering, I found her in the kitchen, visibly agitated.

"I can't find my glasses. They were here just a minute ago." She had removed them to wash her hair and had apparently misplaced them in the process.

There she stood, wet hair dripping on the kitchen floor, along with the tears rolling down her cheeks. I have no idea what came over me in that moment, but when I opened my mouth, "Oh, Mom, it's the disease making you forget," tumbled out.

A split second later I saw a flash of burning rage come into her eyes. Had she been a dragon, I would have been a blackened pile of rubble. "DON'T YOU EVER SAY THAT TO ME AGAIN!" she roared, with every ounce of rage she could muster.

I instantly regretted my choice of words. *What possessed me to say such a thing?* Talk about a lack of empathy and understanding! It was the truth, but so very hurtful for her to hear. I've thought about this incident many times since then. I did not consciously attempt to hurt her, but some deep-seated dragon of my own found its way to the surface. This dragon lashed out at her using hurtful words, in response to the numerous times over the years she had skewered me with her hurtful words. It was the one and only time I mentioned the dreaded word "disease" to Mom. I am humbled by what stress and helplessness can do to a person, on either side of the Alzheimer's fence.

Another afternoon when I arrived at her apartment, Mom proudly announced, "Wait 'til you see what I found!"

She seemed quite excited by something and led me over to her small bookshelf, where she kept framed photographs of family, and on top of which she always saved her week's worth of mail for me to look through. She held up a picture torn out of a magazine of a Latino man standing next to a blond woman, advertising some type of cologne. "I saw this picture of you and Lionel in my magazine and cut it out to show you!" she announced. My husband is Hispanic and my hair is blond, but that photo was not of us.

"Uh, yeah! Wow. Well, thank you, Mom," I exclaimed as I gave her a hug. I didn't know what else to say, and didn't want to burst her bubble by saying it wasn't Lionel and me. Most of the time I found it less stressful for both of us to go along with her odd ideas and strange thoughts, provided they weren't harmful in any way.

While at her apartment on my weekly visits, a certain pattern unfolded, which included fixing her hair, sorting her mail, resetting her answering machine message that mysteriously erased itself on a regular basis, ironing clothes, and any other little chore she wished done.

Once a month, I arranged her pills, which were put in daily by-the-meal pill holders. She was taking more than 19 pills a day, not all of which were prescription. Feeling like an amateur pharmacist, I opened the cupboard in her small kitchen nook, pulled out four empty "Monday through Sunday" weekly pill holders, along with numerous bottles of pills, sat down at her card table with all of it and began to sort and fill. There was calcium (both pills and chewable chocolate squares) for her bones in addition to extra magnesium to help absorb the calcium, glucosamine/chondroitin to help her joints, both vitamin E and folic acid for memory function, vitamin C for immune function, and vitamin B-12 that helped eliminate the tingling sensations in her hands and arms. All these were in addition to her prescription medications. These pills were my (misguided?) effort to promote her "health and vitality." Although it was done with the best of intentions, I now question *why* I had her swallowing so many pills.

By now, in addition to Aricept, she was also taking Namenda, another medication designed to alleviate the symptoms of Alzheimer's disease. Like Aricept, Namenda treats the cognitive symptoms of Alzheimer's by regulating the activity of a chemical messenger (in this case, glutamate) involved with memory and learning. She took a pain medication for her arthritis, the once-a-week (in a perfect world) osteoporosis medication, and an anti-depressant. I often looked at that little, yellow, oblong antidepressant as I placed it in her pillbox and thought to myself, *where were you 50 years ago?*

I had long ago recognized that my mother suffered from depression. By the time my teenage years had arrived, it was very evident to me that I was living with one unhappy woman. For many years, I suffered from delusional thinking that it was somehow my fault that she was so miserable. The screaming and slapping were part and parcel of life in my house. My dad seemed impervious to her tirades. Of course, he managed to escape by being involved in every activity possible. Except for Friday evenings, when Mom had her bowling league, I rarely saw my Dad when I was growing up, and often felt I saw too much of Mom.

In later years, long after I'd grown and left home, I broached the subject of antidepressants with her on more than one occasion. On each of these occasions, I was met with an icy stare and complete denial of her unpleasant behavior. Now that she had dementia, swallowing an antidepressant each day was no longer an issue, and from my perspective, improved her mood.

As Mom's Alzheimer's disease worsened, I realized the

time would come when she would need more skilled care. I decided one of my markers for her needing more active supervision would be when she quit taking her pills properly on her own (excluding the osteoporosis pill, because I was already aware she wasn't taking it only once per week as directed).

We did eventually eliminate the extra magnesium she was taking because it was determined to be causing her consistently loose stools. Stopping these magnesium pills corrected one issue and accorded us a new one, however.

As part of our daily phone call, Mom began complaining, "Vicki, I have to stop eating those tasty little chocolates you give me every day. They're so good, but I can't have them anymore," she stated. Those "tasty chocolates" were chewable calcium squares, which were easy for her to chew, and two less calcium pills to swallow every day.

"Why, Mom?" I couldn't imagine what she was thinking now.

"Well, those little squares go right through me. When I go poop, they drop right out of me, plop, plop, plop."

I muffled my chuckle, "Oh, no, Mom, those little chocolate calcium squares are not coming out of you. Your bowel movements have gotten hard since we stopped the magnesium." I might as well have been talking to the proverbial brick wall, which surely would have understood me better. In the end, it was easier to also discontinue the chewable calcium than to keep explaining every time she had a bowel movement that, no, the chewable calcium was not passing through undigested. The solution? I added yet another pill—a stool softener, which solved the problem of plop, plop, plop.

Mom became agitated every month when the facility bill arrived for their rent plus Dad's nursing care. I did my best to reassure her that all was well, and compliment her about having saved money for this time (although she reminded me each and every time that *this* was not what she had in mind when dutifully adding money to their savings). One never knows what the future holds.

Additional bills or insurance "Explanation of Benefits" for medical care also seemed upsetting to her. While my parents rarely had medical bills to pay outright because of Medicare and private insurance, Mom had trouble deciphering what the sheets of paper said; all she could discern was that it seemed she owed everyone money. It wasn't uncommon for her to throw away the paperwork and proudly present me with the empty envelope she hid and saved for me. After countless rounds of explaining what each letter meant, and her continued inability to comprehend, it became evident the plan we had devised for her to save all the mail in a stack on her table for me to sort through each week had to be changed. In order to shield her from further agitation and eliminate the disappearing paper, I individually called or wrote to change the mailing address to my house for as much of this type of mail as I could.

I am always amazed at how junk mail can find its way to a new address. It seemed as if my parents received solicitations by the truckload. Somehow they appeared to be on every mailing list in the United States, especially those having to do with political agendas and/or charities. The political mail was particularly upsetting to her. These letters all wanted donations: donations to stop illegal immigration, prevent an "imminent war with Mexico," help elect a politician, not to mention the usual appeals from any number of social or medical organizations, as well as advocacy groups for senior citizens. Most of the rhetoric in these solicitations did nothing but upset her.

"I didn't sleep a wink last night. I am so worried about the war."

"What war?" I asked her. *Was Mom really that astute about the Iraq war?*

"You know!" she replied, "the war we will be having with Mexico! I just don't feel like I can send them any money to help stop it, though."

I did my best to reassure her there wasn't going to be a war with Mexico in the near future, and she didn't need to worry about sending them money. Most of these solicitations caused no end to her grief, because she felt she could not afford to help defend her country. Having grown up in a small town comprised almost exclusively of people of northern European descent in a time when people of any color other than white were considered inferior, my parents were very prejudiced. While I was sometimes disturbed by some of the "non-politically correct" comments or words that came out of my parents' mouths, I felt I could not personally hold them responsible, as they were only acting and speaking in a manner that reflected the time and place where they grew up.

I repeatedly wrote letters and made phone calls, requesting these organizations remove my parents' names from their mailing lists. As the appeal letters continued to arrive on a regular basis, I sometimes felt frustrated by the bureaucracy, but it didn't discourage me in my quest to eliminate this junk mail from my mother's life. It took almost two years, but gratefully, it finally ceased, and I felt like throwing a party to celebrate!

Changing the mailing address for the vast majority of Mom's mail reduced her stress on one level, but on another level represented one more loss for her. It was clear to me that collecting the mail was an important part of each resident's daily routine, judging by the crowd of people with post office box keys that gathered near the facility mailboxes each afternoon. It was something to look forward to, because who knew what interesting item of mail might appear? Sadly, the mail in Mom's box diminished to a trickle of inane form letters and advertisements. Nevertheless, she still went to collect her mail on a daily basis, hoping for what, I do not know.

For the first couple of years at Cedar Grove, my mother, the meticulous housekeeper, continued to do an adequate job of keeping her apartment clean. It was only as time progressed that evidence of her cognitive decline became apparent through her lack of cleanliness.

Although she had a small stackable washer and dryer unit in her apartment, she found it easier to take her sheets and towels to the larger washing machine in the common laundry room down the hall from her apartment. This highlights Mom's steely determination to remain independent. Somehow, she managed to carry her sheets and towels with arthritic hands, while limping on arthritic legs, down the long hallway to the laundry room, and later back again with her freshly laundered linens. Occasionally, she also stayed to do her ironing in the communal laundry room on a full-size ironing board, rather than the compact travel-size ironing board in her apartment. Even though irons were available in the common laundry room, she preferred to bring her own. After her iron went missing, however, this shared laundry room became her only choice for ironing until I began to do it for her.

"Somebody stole my iron," Mom told me one day when I called.

"What? Really?" I didn't know what to say. *Why would someone steal an iron?*

"Yes, somebody came into my apartment when I wasn't here and stole my iron, right out of my dresser drawer."

"Hmm. Well, we'll have to track it down when I come to see you this week, okay?"

When I visited that week, I searched every nook and cranny of her apartment, as well as both the communal laundry rooms, and asked the facility caregivers to keep an eye out for an errant iron. We never did find out what happened to her iron, but I now suspect Mom either left it in the main laundry room, and someone took it to their room and forgot to bring it back, or Mom loaned it to someone and that person forgot from whom she had borrowed it. It will always remain one of those great, unsolved mysteries.

Mom, on the other hand, never gave up on her story that someone came into her apartment and "stole it." It was this sometimes blind faith in Mom that eventually triggered a conflict between the facility administrator and me. Mom was my mother and there was a part of me that wanted to believe her. It's obvious to me now that I did not yet have a complete grasp of dementia, and how it was wreaking havoc in my mother's brain.

Other items "disappeared" as well, including a book I'd written detailing our family's history, and all her lovely jewelry. Over the years, Mom's aunt had given her several pairs of elegant earrings as gifts. I especially remember the Mount St. Helen earrings Mom told me would be mine someday. I had always admired the bright, green gemstone created from the ash of that mountain's volcanic eruption in 1980. Mom also had at least two pairs of Black Hills Gold earrings from her aunt, and a set of expensive pearl earrings and necklace Dad gave her for their 30th wedding anniversary. All these and more had simply vanished. I have come to believe she probably put them inside a container of some kind and threw it away when she was "cleaning." Mom did love to have a place for all things and put all things in their place.

One day when I came to visit, Mom proudly stated, "I've done some cleaning this week." Something in the way she said the word "cleaning" put me on instant alert. I was filled with mild trepidation, as I thought to myself, *oh no, what has she thrown away now?* She brought out her wallet and opened it to show me that it contained $15 and nothing else. She had thrown away all her and Dad's insurance cards, her state ID card, the Medicare cards, and several other identity cards for various organizations. The things that don't occur to caregivers (me) until they happen! I did my best not to lose my cool even though there was a part of me that wanted to scream. Luckily, after digging through all her trashcans, which thankfully hadn't been emptied yet, I found a few of the cards/ID's. Over the next week, I spent several hours on the phone tracking down new cards for the ones not found.

The story didn't end there, however, as even though I believed I'd looked everywhere in her apartment for the missing cards, in my stressed-out state of mind I'd obviously overlooked a small green canister buried underneath clothing in the back of her closet. Imagine my surprise when cleaning her closet several weeks later, uncovering this canister, opening it, and coming face to face with the rest of the missing ID cards! Looking on the bright side, this meant we now had duplicates of the cards—just in case.

Each week after the various chores were done, we were off to "tea time" with Dad in The Cottage. Because my father is not talkative, tea time was a good time to arrive because we could all participate. We enjoyed coffee or tea, and some sort of cookie or cake together at the dining table. The remainder of the time we'd watch TV in Dad's room, or Mom would shave Dad.

Throughout my life, I have always been closer to my mother than my father. She was the "communicator," he, the quiet one. Engaging him in a conversation normally resulted in grunts and smiles on his part, but few words. Over the years, I can remember very few meaningful conversations with him. With his Parkinson's disease and growing dementia, it became a creative challenge for me to find ways to interface with him. Touch is important to all humans, and he was no exception, so it soon became the avenue through which we could connect. He liked to hold hands, and I think he also enjoyed the human touch involved in trimming his hair, as that was one of the few questions he'd ask me on a regular basis.

"Doesn't my hair need a trim?"

"Not yet, Dad, I just trimmed it last week."

"Oh, okay, maybe next week?"

"Yes, maybe next week."

One of the less-pleasant aspects of care that involved "touch" was trimming his toenails. It involved handling his smelly feet, and I will be the first to admit that I tended to put off this task for as long as possible. His nails were yellow, thick, brittle, and difficult to trim, even after first soaking them in a plastic tub of water. I did this for two years before learning that there was a podiatrist who came to the facility every few months to trim toenails, and Medicare even covered the procedure. Trimming my father's toenails was a task I happily (and right there on the spot) gave up—no one had to ask me twice.

By 4:30, I usually made my good-byes, with hugs and kisses for each of them. Normally when I left The Cottage, the two of them were either sitting in Dad's room watching television, or were in his bathroom together completely engrossed in shaving his face, despite the fact that the staff had already shaved him that morning.

"Hold still!" Mom sternly commanded.

"Ouch, you are scraping my face!" Dad spoke sharply as I gingerly walked out of his bedroom with a sigh, shaking my head and thinking to myself, *some things never change.*

My step was brisk as I approached The Cottage exit, pushing the appropriate button code next to the door that flashed a green light, signaling that it was safe to open the door to "freedom" without setting off an alarm. Occasionally, a resident stood by the door waiting and hoping someone might come along and open the door so they could leave too. It was at times like this that I felt like I was exiting a prison, which in a way, I suppose I was, although the real prison for these residents was their own minds.

Guilt always walked out this door with me; I never managed to leave it behind. After arriving home, I often phoned one of my children because it felt therapeutic for me to hear someone speak who had plans and dreams for tomorrow. This also helped me to mask the ever-present worry, real or imagined, that I was not doing more, being more, and giving more to my parents.

Each evening I made a point of calling Mom to check on her and hear her litany of complaints about everything in her and Dad's life, in addition to the shortcomings of the facility. My daily calls to her went on for nearly three years, as much as possible, even if I was out of town or out of the country. In the end, this was neither a good nor a healthy idea. It became a sort of ball and chain for both of us, more stressful than helpful. As time went on, Mom had greater difficulty forming coherent sentences, which was stressful for her, and I had difficulty straining to decipher them, often playing a version of "20 Questions," in my attempt to figure out what she was trying to say.

Lessons Learned

Do not remind your loved one she is losing her memory, and try to avoid using words like "disease." This seems simple enough, but when experiencing stress, I believe it's common for our tongues to get ahead of our brains.

Do not confront or question the memory of the person suffering from dementia in any of its forms. Playing along with his or her fantasy is less stressful for everyone. If necessary, you can check out the facts later with the facility.

Exercise compassion—practice responding to and empathizing with your loved-one's feelings, rather than his or her often accusatory or angry words. Remember how frightening life must be for him or her at times.

Guilt is real and probably unavoidable. If you treat your loved one the way you would want him or her to treat you, you are doing the best you can and who could ask more? When you are together, find joy in small things, such as a smile or holding hands. This time will not last forever. Also remember to take time for yourself to renew and re-charge, away from your loved one.

Be aware that a person with memory loss may "accidentally" throw away important papers or valuable belongings. It is better to unobtrusively remove important papers/ID cards than have to replace them. If necessary, return copies for your loved one's files. Some valuables (such as Mom's jewelry) are irreplaceable.

Find out which services are covered by Medicare or offered by the facility that might help make your life easier (for me it was toenail care), and arrange for your loved one to receive them.

Be careful not to set up routines out of guilt (for me it was daily phone calls) that become a ball and chain for both you and your loved one. Join a support group where you can vent your guilt and let it go.

SIXTEEN
Decline

With each passing week my mother's writing skills decreased, until it became necessary for me to do all the writing for her—everything from bill-paying to writing birthday cards to her grandkids. Sadly, her severely arthritic fingers could no longer coordinate this motor skill, which consequently also put an end to her habitual list-making of things she needed done, or things she wanted to tell me (normally a list of complaints). Mom's inability to write became one more item on the growing list of ways she was losing control over her life. Dad had already faced this loss and didn't seem bothered by it. Mom didn't take loss nearly as well. I also noted that word retrieval was becoming more problematic as Mom sometimes struggled to find the right word during conversations with me.

Another list Mom always kept was for items she "needed" from the store, which often included facial tissues. Both she and my dad were happiest when they had at least three or more tissues in their pockets. My dad actually liked to carry one in his hand, smoothing it out or folding it up over and over again, probably as a form of much-needed tactile stimulation.

Sometime over the course of the first year following my parents' move, Mom's escalating paranoia became evident as she began accusing me of stealing her money on a regular basis. Looking back, I am sure this was a control, or better said, loss-of-control, issue. Paranoia is a common occurrence with people who have dementia. I didn't recognize this at first, and took her behavior quite personally.

Her accusatory behavior dragged on for a very long time. In the beginning, I was still operating under the assumption that the woman in front of me was my mother as I had always known her—her accusations brought me to tears and spurred proclamations of my innocence. Whenever a phone call started with, "I'm so disgusted," her voice a deep whisper, my heart sank, and I knew it was not going to be a good conversation. She would then proceed to talk about me in the third person, "I am so disgusted with my daughter." Of course, I consistently took the bait and said, "Why?" Her reply was usually something along the lines of, "Well, she married a dirty Mexican, and they are using my money to travel." Of course there were always variations on this theme when she became angry with me, and I never quite knew what accusation would spill out of her mouth. I always attempted to reason with her, but to no avail. Early on, I argued, defended, cajoled, cried, or inevitably raised my voice in disagreement. Though it took quite a long time, eventually I realized these responses only served to infuriate or devastate her. It was more productive to either attempt to redirect the conversation or, if that didn't work, just listen until she wound down, then change the subject.

At the same time, she developed a liking for my brother, and enjoyed it immensely when he occasionally called her.

I moved all their paperwork files to my house because I felt I could no longer trust her to keep from throwing away important papers. Thus, when she started accusing me of "stealing" her money, I felt the need to show her the blatant truth, supported by undeniable, hardcopy evidence. This entailed gathering and bringing all the files containing bank statements, investment summaries, and bill receipts back to her apartment to prove my innocence. Once, when I arrived at her apartment with all the paperwork in hand, my dad was waiting with her. She had him present beside her as a "show of force" to help prove my guilt and to "bring me to justice." The best part of this meeting was when Dad, in a totally lucid, and unexpected moment, stated, "We should be appreciating all she does for us. I think you should be thanking her instead of making all these accusations." Well, that certainly took the wind out of her sails! Naturally, her retort was the usual indignant, "Well, I am always wrong. I might as well go jump off a bridge." I was used to my mother saying this. It has been typical of her for as long as I can remember. All I could do was shrug my shoulders and move on.

These accusations recurred with some frequency, and I don't even know why I continued to carefully collect and bring the paperwork to her, as she no longer understood the bank statements and investment summaries anyway. In retrospect, I suspect it was more for me, still attempting to prove to my mother that I was a "good girl."

It was always difficult and hurtful to be accused of stealing my parents' money, even if I knew Mom's accusations were a result of dementia. My well-intentioned goal was to stretch their money as far as possible by spending it judiciously, calling upon the frugality I learned from both my parents. Again, my reactionary behavior came as a result of the fact that I wasn't yet fully grasping what Alzheimer's does to a person. If a person has a rather negative personality trait, it seems Alzheimer's disease often takes that trait and magnifies it. I simply wasn't prepared for this.

Even though I knew my mother had Alzheimer's disease, in the first few years I didn't assimilate what that meant. I felt I had educated myself on this deplorable disease through books and medical pamphlets shared with me by my local chapter of the Alzheimer's Association, but somehow I didn't perceive the brain changes that were occurring in my parents, and most markedly in my mother. Maybe it was because my mother and I were in a sort of denial phase, but looking back, I believe I could have handled situations better had I been able to more fully understand what was happening to her cognitive processes. Time and again, her disease proved to be not only a journey for her, but for me as well.

I think I could have saved myself plenty of tears, lost sleep, agitation, anxiety, and heartache if I had only arrived sooner at the place of acceptance where I now reside. I learned how to take loving care of these people who were but mere shadows of the parents I once knew, remembering that they were demented and not the people I once knew. They may have existed in our world, but they were not of it.

Eventually, I learned to distance myself from my mother's hurtful comments and no longer take them personally. I could listen to her, but cease reacting or agonizing over the things she said. I need not argue, reason, confront, or make any attempt to convince her she was wrong! It didn't matter any longer. What mattered were my parents' feelings, accepting Mom and Dad as they were, and loving them despite their disabilities. This was easier said than done, however, as I can attest to in my journey. The sooner a caregiver reaches this place of acceptance, the less pain and angst he or she will experience.

My mother always wielded great control over me, and my sense of guilt is perhaps over-developed as a result. I am amazed at how much guilt I felt over trivial events and occurrences. *Should I be calling more often? Should I be visiting more often, maybe every day? What could I bring them to make their life happier?* More and more I felt responsible for my parents' happiness. After all, I had been instrumental in moving them away from their lifetime home. I continued to be plagued by insomnia, my brain working overtime in an attempt to devise ways to make their lives more interesting and comfortable, and yes, more meaningful. What can a person who no longer writes, reads, or understands television or books on tape because the brain doesn't process the information well even do with such a short attention span? What if this person also cannot walk (or at least not very well), so getting out and about is difficult? Listening to music was dependent upon the caregiver's time schedule because my parents were unable to operate anything mechanical, and when I suggested this activity, they both appeared ambivalent. *What could they do to pass the time?* I felt grateful for any activities organized by the facility in which they were able to participate.

This brings me to my thoughts on the name "assisted living facilities." Assisted living facilities might be more appropriately called "assisted waiting facilities," because it's my observation that residents in these facilities are "waiting," whether it's waiting to pass on, waiting for something to finally happen, or just waiting for the next meal, help getting into their bed, or using the toilet. I'm not sure how much "living" is going on, as it appears to be more of an existence than a life. Yes, I realize "assisted living" has a much more positive connotation, and I can be accused of being cynical, but my opinion is based upon what I witnessed with my own eyes. Maybe it showcases the whole idea in a positive light so those of us with family members in assisted living facilities can more easily swallow our guilt for not caring for them at home. In a different time or place, most of these elderly people would have already passed on, or if not, would be cared for in a relative's home.

We have outsmarted ourselves with our medical technology; we've achieved the ability to keep people alive past their time of feeling like an active, contributing member of society. I do not judge, I only comment on what I observe. I have talked to many people about this "existence," and have yet to find anyone who wishes it for him or herself. I'm left wondering why we think our parents, spouses, or other family members would want to be kept alive with fortified drinks, handfeeding by a caregiver, or worse, feeding tubes. To my knowledge, people with Alzheimer's disease are not going to suddenly have symptoms disappear, regain their former selves, and be able to leave the facility to lead a normal life again. I'm not suggesting euthanasia, but I am suggesting we consciously consider *our* motivations when faced with these interventions. Mom made it very clear to me many times that she did not wish to live in this manner, so I had no illusions about what she wanted if that time eventually came for her.

Think over this example—the facility called each autumn to tell me, "The nurse is at the facility giving flu shots. Would you like us to give your parents flu shots?" The first three years I answered without thinking, *of course* I wanted them to have a flu shot. What kind of daughter would I be if I denied them this medical intervention to "protect" them from the flu? After a time, I began to analyze why I instinctively always answered, "Yes" without actually thinking about what I was affirming. Didn't flu shots fall into the same "grey" preventative health care area as vitamins? By the fourth year when the facility called me to ask about the flu shot, I said, "No." In response, I received a somewhat incredulous "You don't want them to have a flu shot?" I tried not to let this statement and its underlying accusation affect me, but I couldn't help the fact that it dredged up those same deep-seated feelings of guilt. I wanted to do what was best for my parents, and I had to remind myself to not feel contrite for trying to honor their wishes. Battling the guilt was an ongoing process. While I don't know if it's something I will ever be able to fully let go, I know I continued to examine their "quality of life," honored their wishes, and made decisions accordingly.

Lessons Learned

As your loved one's reasoning and writing skills diminish, you will acquire the bill-paying responsibilities. In order for this to be feasible, it will be necessary to list your name on all checking/savings accounts, credit card accounts, telephone, TV, utility services, or any other bills/accounts so that you can sign the checks, and/or interface with any customer service representatives, if needed.

Don't take it personally if a loved one suffering from dementia acts out negatively towards you, displays paranoid or accusatory behavior, or anything of the like. Remember that a negative personality trait often becomes more severe with the progression of Alzheimer's, and paranoia is a common characteristic manifested in Alzheimer's patients.

I learned to accept my parents as they were—dementia and all—and realized how important it was to remain calm and quiet in most situations rather than reason, defend, argue, or cajole. Insisting I was right only created disharmony. Learning to accept the blame graciously (even when you're not to blame) can avoid an angry confrontation, which serves no constructive purpose for anyone involved. Smother your own ego! Some days will be better than others. Delight in those good days.

Fight the guilt when it comes to medical interventions! No matter what caregivers or others might think about your actions, remember what your loved ones' wishes are, and honor them guilt-free—after all, you're doing what your loved one expressly wanted.

SEVENTEEN
Anger, Shavers and Infidelity

While Mom continued to direct her anger toward me, it soon overflowed and spread to my father's caregivers as well. She considered it her duty to not only spend all day, every day, sitting with my father, but to continue to attend to the one thing she felt she could still do for him each day: shaving his face with an electric razor.

Unfortunately, she took it to the extreme, often spending 45 or more minutes at this task. It was hard on my dad's skin, but he loved being touched by her, so he endured it. As a result, his skin became very red and irritated; my mother then continually complained about his red skin, not understanding that she was, in fact, the cause of it. Different caregivers tried hiding the shaver from her, but she put up such a fuss that in the end, they gave it back to her. I brought Dad some soothing aftershave, but I'm not sure how often someone patted it on his abused facial skin.

Sometimes, my father actually told her he didn't want to be shaved that particular day. She then pouted and carried on with her usual "I might as well go jump in the river" talk, so either way, he suffered. The day she shaved off his bushy white eyebrows was the last straw for one caregiver. Mom rushed to the phone to tell me, "That damn caregiver took away your Dad's shaver, and threw it across the room and broke it. Vicki, you have no idea how mean these people are! It's simply atrocious how they treat us and on top of that, now I've no way to shave your dad." I was skeptical of this report, yet impressed she came up with the word "atrocious." I patiently listened to her litany of complaints about the caregiver's so-called wicked behavior. I later learned it was she who had thrown the shaver across the room when confronted by the staff about Dad's missing eyebrows. This was an example of her ability to twist her own actions around and blame them on someone else. For the longest time, I more or less believed what she told me on the phone every night when I dutifully called to say hello and ask about her day. I imagined that there was a possibility that whatever she was telling me could have happened, and since she was my mother, I gave her the benefit of the doubt.

It wasn't uncommon for her to call and say, "I'm so mad at your father. I spent all day with him and he didn't say two words to me. When I asked him who I am, he said 'I don't know.' Can you believe that? After all I have done for him, he says he doesn't know who I am!" Incensed, she would say, "Well, he can just stew in his own juices because I am not going to visit him anymore." This resulted in her "punishing" him by not visiting for a few days. Instead of going to see him in The Cottage, she'd sit in her apartment and brood about how poorly he'd treated her, which caused her no end of tears and more uncontrolled scratching. Whether her skin condition was caused by nervousness, dermatitis, or a combination thereof, emotional upsets were apt to cause her to obessively scratch at her skin. It gave the appearance she had fleas, and I am sure it was painful, especially when she scratched the skin raw and it bled. Doctors found no definitive cause, so we continually tried different lotions to soothe her skin.

When she was upset by something Dad did or didn't do, she often told me she lay awake all night crying. How very, very sad this was for her. He, on the other hand, had absolutely no clue why she wasn't visiting. Because time seems different for people with dementia, I'm not sure he even realized she wasn't visiting him. Other times when she visited, he begged her to stay and sleep with him.

Chuckling, she'd tell me, "Oh, Vicki, your dad is something else. Today when I was ready to leave, he begged me *again* to stay over and sleep with him tonight. Isn't that the funniest thing? I told him, 'Harry, there is barely room for you in that tiny bed. Where do you think you'd put me?'"

One of the caregivers occasionally brought her baby son to the facility on her days off for the residents to hold and enjoy, which was quite thoughtful of her. On one such day, my mother saw my dad holding this caregiver's baby, and subsequently called me to say, "Well, your dad's son came to visit him today."

"Huh?" was my confused reply. *That's odd. Did Jack fly in for an impromptu visit without telling me?*

Mom then went on in an accusatory manner, "Yeah, I think he's having an affair with that Indian girl, and now she has a baby by your dad. Whenever she comes here, she's always letting Harry hold him, so that's how I know."

Whoa, wait a minute here, I thought to myself, *what's going on?* "Uh, Mom, seriously, I don't think that's possible, but I'll check into it when I come visit, okay?" She seemed willing to accept that, and went on to other complaints.

Somehow I managed to keep a straight face when she continued to talk about it on subsequent visits. My dad was 93 years old at the time, confined to a wheelchair, and rarely lucid. Dementia was the only explanation for my prejudiced mother's belief that my father cheated on her by having an affair with his American Indian caregiver. It might have been funny, if it wasn't so sad.

Mom did not let go of the issue of my dad's "affair" for months, and whenever it came into her mind, she "punished" Dad in her typical manner by not visiting him for a few days. Still, he had no clue what was going on. Mom *often* remembered things we all wished she would forget.

119

Dementia, and specifically Alzheimer's disease, is a devastating disease in so many different ways. It was sometimes hard for me to wrap my mind around, as it affected my parents in such vastly diverse ways.

Soon the food at the facility became an issue for Mom. Unfortunately, the great chef left Cedar Grove for a different job within a couple of months of my parents' arrival, and the meals were never the same again, at least according to Mom. "I don't know where the hell they found that new cook, but he *can't* cook! I think they went out and picked up some guy off the street and said, 'you want a job cooking for old people?' The food has gotten just awful. I've half a mind to just quit going down there for meals and fix something in my room." Incidentally, this past year, that same chef was voted our state's "Chef of the Year" for his consecutively outstanding meals at Cedar Grove. Whenever I joined my parents for a meal at Cedar Grove, I always found that the food tasted fine. In fact, I would go so far as to say it was delicious. Now, I realize her ideas about food and her palate were already beginning to change.

Lesson Learned

Our taste buds become less sensitive as we age, or may be influenced by medications, so perceptions regarding food may be different for the elderly. Complaints may not always be 100 percent valid, but they are certainly worth checking into.

EIGHTEEN
Practicing Patience

I do believe some of my mother's complaints were legitimate. It quickly became apparent that there was little privacy for my father in The Cottage. The lack of privacy would have been unbearable for my mother had she lived in that part of the building.

There were certain requirements for living in The Cottage; like summer camp, each resident needed all personal belongings to be labeled, including clothing, sheets, and towels. Unfortunately, labeling did not rule out the possibility of items disappearing. Within a few weeks, both sets of my dad's new sheets had disappeared, along with most of his towels, and all but two pairs of mismatched socks. One day he had no sheets on his bed when Mom arrived to visit him. She was outraged, to put it mildly. I must admit I was also irritated by the seeming lack of respect given to a resident's belongings.

During my next visit to Cedar Grove, my mother and I stopped by the administrator's office to voice our concerns about my father's missing items. Mary, the administrator, agreed with us that the facility was responsible for the items, so they replaced my dad's towels and socks with new ones, and found alternate sheets for his bed. Upon arrival in Dad's room one subsequent afternoon, Mom noticed his sheets were missing yet again (this time they were only being laundered); she hastily (and brazenly, I am sure) went back to her apartment and brought him her sheets, which were not labeled. By the time I found out about it, *her* sheets had also gone missing. The facility found a used pair of sheets, which they gave her, temporarily smoothing her ruffled feathers. This sheet drama only added more fuel to both her ever-growing list of complaints and my stress level.

It's unfortunate that more care is not given to the residents' belongings, but I surmise that given the mental state of a large percentage of Cottage residents, *they* couldn't care less! This is another example of the loss of control over one's life that residents and their families must undergo. My mother took it very hard, as I can imagine I might in the same situation. She didn't appreciate it when my father turned up in clothes she didn't recognize. It certainly didn't bother him, but she was *not* pleased when his clothing vanished, and someone else's appeared in his closet or on his person.

Another valid complaint was in the way Dad was dressed. He was unable to dress himself, so he had to rely on whatever the caregivers found in his closet on any given day. One cold winter's day, Mom called to tell me, "Vicki, those Cottage workers have no common sense. When I went to see your dad, they had him dressed in a short-sleeved summer shirt! I let them know in no uncertain terms that was not acceptable. He was shivering!" I don't know if they dressed him that way because his warmer clothing was in the laundry, or the caregivers didn't think about him being cold, or perhaps didn't care, but it was certain to provoke Mom's ire.

With The Cottage always seeming short on staff, Dad often had to wait longer than he could for help in going to the bathroom, and before long was put in disposable underwear for those times he couldn't wait. Over time, he became almost completely incontinent. He often wished to lie down, and would wait patiently at his bed for a caregiver to transfer him. I'm sure sitting in a wheelchair for hours a day must grow uncomfortable, and who can blame him for wanting a couple of hours of respite lying on his bed? I know some days the caregivers never did come to his room to help him to bed for an afternoon nap. They were so understaffed and overworked they could not be in three places at once. I am appreciative that there were caregivers at all, but with residents like those in The Cottage needing so much extra care, it was unfortunate there weren't enough.

It was not unusual to find someone else in my father's bed, or to find my father in someone else's room attempting to get into his or her bed. The rooms, clothes, and beds all seemed interchangeable. It scared Mom when she came to see him and found a strange woman in his bed, or a man sitting in his room looking lost. Occasionally, someone attempted to crawl into my dad's bed when he was already in it. Such was life in The Cottage.

My mother's complaints about the food, the caregivers, the room temperature, Dad's clothing, and the way my dad "behaved" went on without end in nearly every conversation I had with her. I did my best to follow up on her complaints because I wanted to please her and take good care of the two of them, but after more than two years of this, I grew weary, dreading our daily call. Sadly, though, I found that not calling each day made her even angrier and more difficult to interact with when we did talk.

Whenever I traveled out of town, she became sullen and angry, and sometimes would react even more negatively towards me than usual. Of course, there was always the accompanying accusation that I was stealing their money to take these trips. She was suspicious that Lionel was not really a physician who earned a good living, and suggested that I lied about his profession to cover up the fact that I was stealing their money. The reason I know this was because she told several of the administrative staff at Cedar Grove her "suspicions," which were then passed along to me. I tried not telling her when we went out of town, but invariably, a situation would arise where she or Dad needed something, which resulted in a confession from me that I wasn't in town. This caused more anger and hurt feelings that I hadn't told her we were leaving. I couldn't seem to win.

Soon general accusations began to run rampant. I knocked on her door one Thursday afternoon, and when she opened the door, I could see by the look on her face that this was going to be a difficult afternoon. I decided to ignore her foul mood and overcompensate by being especially sweet. As always, I washed her hair, rolled it up in curlers and dried it with her hand-held hairdryer. There was little conversation until she suddenly blurted out, "You never take me anywhere." I looked at her with incredulity.

"Mom, I ask you every week if you'd like to go out. You always tell me no!"

She continued, "Besides that, what good would it do if you did take me out?   You won't give me any spending money. What have you done with all my money?   Traveled with it, and enjoyed spending it, I don't doubt."

Of course I had given her "spending" money whenever she told me she had "no money." Sometimes I thought she might have put the money in an envelope for "safekeeping" that eventually ended up in the trash, so imagine my surprise when I later found more than $140 in an empty medicine bottle! I learned where it all went—nowhere! I think it gave her a momentary sense of control to see that money and know she could spend it if she wished. Unfortunately, in her current life, there were not many opportunities to spend money.

During this time, I reflected on all my parents had to let go of, especially my mother, and how very difficult it was to leave all that was familiar and comfortable behind. She had already lost the familiarity of her physical surroundings by leaving her lifetime home, and was now in the process of losing her mental capacities. Comments, such as "I can't remember anything anymore," or "I've lost my mind," made it apparent she realized her mental acuity was failing. It must have been terrifying for her.

The primary family member caregiver has many roles to play, but none are more important than sharing time, patience, and loving forgiveness. If the caregiver is an adult child as I was, part of the journey is the realization that these people are no longer the parents we once knew, but some aberration of their former selves. Time and attention for these fragile people, even if it is just sitting and holding their hands, is so important.

Throughout the journey, I continued to yearn for an involved sibling, someone to share the burden and help maneuver the often-bumpy road. Although it was disappointing for me to not have my brother's active support, my parents still needed caring for, whether or not he chose to be engaged. Clearly, it is helpful and undoubtedly less stressful if there is sibling interaction and support.

Lessons Learned

Let go of preconceived expectations if your loved one is living in an assisted-living or care facility. As long as they wear appropriate, clean clothing and have clean sheets on his/her bed, accept that he/she may not necessarily be sleeping in his/her own sheets or wearing his/her own clothes. If it isn't bothering him/her, don't let it bother you. Do keep valuable items, such as burial clothing or expensive jewelry, in a safe place outside of the facility. My dad's white dress shirt disappeared from his closet before I realized I should have brought his suit and shirt to my house for safekeeping.

Be as sensitive as possible to the many losses someone with dementia, and particularly an Alzheimer's patient, is experiencing. Most of the time it is probably better to be open and upfront, even if you run the risk of hurt feelings. Trying to hide information will ultimately backfire as it did for me when I would leave town and not tell Mom.

Keep reminding yourself that your loved one with dementia is not the person you once knew, but he or she still needs loving kindness and understanding. Practice patience and never discount the power of touch.

NINETEEN
Nearly Vaporized

My parents had lived at Cedar Grove for nearly 15 months when I began noticing that Mary James, the administrator, seemed rather distant in my presence. When we interacted, I sensed a certain curtness and irritability that I did not observe in her interactions with other visitors. I made an attempt to not personalize it, deciding instead she was only busy or otherwise distracted. Looking back, however, an incident that occurred between us makes me think it was more than simple distraction or stress that caused her cool aloofness toward me.

The "incident" occurred around the time that Cedar Grove informed me all bubble-wrapped medications had to be ordered from and processed by a particular pharmacy because Cedar Grove had a new contract with this pharmacy. This pharmacy was contracted to print out a monthly med sheet or "MAR," bubble-wrap (securing individual pills inside little plastic bubbles to make counting and administering them easier for the caregivers), and provide the medications for everyone in The Cottage, including Dad. I was informed that the pharmacy I had been using could not provide the necessary paperwork, so I conformed to the new rules, and Dad's medications now came from the new pharmacy.

Up until this time, I had personally picked up and delivered my father's bubble-wrapped prescriptions, along with his OTC medications, from another pharmacy. I had originally confirmed with Cedar Grove's staff nurse that this arrangement was satisfactory. However, I later learned that behind my back, that same staff nurse told the administrator I was "difficult."

The reason I had purchased Dad's meds from a different pharmacist, coincidentally also a friend of mine, was because she charged less for meds and the bubble-wrap than Cedar Grove's "preferred" pharmacy. Evidently, by delivering Dad's meds, I made it more difficult for the Cedar Grove nurses to track his prescriptions, so I was perceived to be difficult. My attempt to be frugal with my parents' money irritated the Cedar Grove nurse because it inconvenienced her.

Only a couple of months later, I learned from my original pharmacist that she could now supply the needed MAR paperwork, bubble-wrapping at a lesser cost, plus free delivery to Cedar Grove. I was pleased to hear this. This pharmacist had been disappointed because there were other residents at the Cedar Grove facility that had also previously received their prescription medications from her, and she had lost several longtime customers because of the new program.

The very same afternoon I learned this new information from my pharmacist friend, I arrived at the facility to visit my parents, and happened to notice the administrator in the lobby. I was so excited by the thought of helping my pharmacist friend, not to mention that I could save my dad and other residents money, that I threw caution to the wind and decided to tell the administrator all about it. "Mary, guess what? Dad's former pharmacist can now do everything that the other pharmacy can do, like print the MAR, bubble wrap, and deliver meds to the facility at no cost!"

She nodded and said, "Yes, we heard."

"Oh, that's great! Have you been able to tell her other former customers here they now have a choice?"

The administrator glared at me and said curtly, "We only found this out earlier today. Obviously, we haven't told anyone about it yet."

I had the feeling that my effort to help out my pharmacist friend had somehow backfired. Before I could extract one foot from my mouth, I was about to stick in the other one.

As the administrator continued glaring at me, another resident's daughter, whom I knew, walked up to the front desk where we were standing. The administrator said, "Sandra, we took your mom to The Cottage yesterday."

Sandra replied, "You did? How'd she do?"

Stressed and not thinking clearly, I completely misinterpreted what was happening when I looked at Sandra and blurted out, "They took your mom to The Cottage without telling you?" This was not a good choice of words.

This appeared to be the last straw for the administrator, as it was apparent from her brittle voice that I'd said completely the wrong thing. "*Of course* we didn't just take her mother to The Cottage," she spit out the words like a machine gun.

Then Sandra turned to me and said, "It was just a practice run to see how she'd do, as she'll soon be needing to move there."

Now I understood; I had misinterpreted. But it was too late in the eyes of the administrator. I felt her eyes bore holes in me as she proceeded to inform me, "You know, Vicki, you often come across as suspicious of the care here, and what just happened is a prime example. Why is that? The staff nurse told me you are difficult to work with, and personally, I think you are too emotional when visiting our facility. Besides that," her tirade continued, "you've no right to stand here, and offend and insult other residents' families!"

If I could have melted into a puddle, I would have. I felt blindsided by her outburst, and did what I naturally do when someone lashes out at me; I began crying. This all happened in front of everyone in the lobby. I was absolutely mortified, and I thought Sandra looked mortified as well. I wished I were a turtle in that moment, so that I could have sought refuge within the safety of my own shell.

When I started to cry, the administrator pulled me into her office where she continued to berate me with a litany of my shortcomings. Finally, I couldn't handle it any longer, and told her point blank, "I can't listen to this anymore. I'm done listening to you." I believe this would be referred to as the "fight or flight response." Considering how averse I am to confrontation, flight seemed the best option at the moment. Her parting words were "come back and talk when you aren't so emotional." I would rather face a firing squad, I thought to myself as I rushed out of her office.

I pulled myself together as I walked up the three flights of stairs to my mother's apartment, but was feeling devastated by the administrator's remarks. Would it not have been more professional to set up a time with me in private to air her concerns? I didn't care if I ever talked to this woman again. I started to dream of moving my parents somewhere else at that very moment, although it would be another year and many tears (not just my tears) before it happened.

When the yearly survey letter from Cedar Grove's corporate office arrived several months later, I sent a personal letter describing my "less than professional" experiences with the administrator, along with the survey to the home office in another state. I received no reply.

The administrator and I didn't speak again until the week my parents moved out of Cedar Grove the following year. I analyzed what she meant by her cutting words. I wrote a letter to her (never mailed), which was my therapy to process the incident. That fateful day in her office, she accused me of being suspicious, difficult, and emotional. She was probably correct on all three counts. Maybe it was her sharp delivery that hurt so badly.

Was I "suspicious?" Well, all I could think of was that my inquiries on behalf of my mother about her fears and her suspicions that people were "stealing" my father's clothing, towels, and bedding implied that I shared those same fears and suspicions. Mom was also convinced the caregivers were not brushing Dad's teeth or shaving him. For her sake, I had spoken with the caregivers, and even had them put up a chart showing they had done these tasks so Mom could see it. Given what Mom was telling me, this request seemed reasonable. Maybe they weren't shaving him or brushing his teeth. How was I to know for sure? Did this make me "suspicious?"

Was I "difficult?" This comment went back to the fact that I wanted to work "outside the box" when dealing with my father's prescription medications. In my attempts to be a "good girl," and use my parents' money wisely, I came across as a "difficult girl."

Was I "emotional?" This accusation was the most surprising to me. Who would NOT be emotional in the situation I was in, with two parents failing before my very eyes? I was so upset by this encounter that I called Sandra, the woman whose mother was taken to The Cottage for a trial run that day, and asked her if I had offended or insulted her. She was quite perplexed by my question, and said she had understood what I meant, and of course she was not offended or insulted. She did tell me she was feeling quite "emotional" over the changes in her mother, and the fact they would soon be moving her into The Cottage because of her Alzheimer's and cognitive decline. We both agreed that we felt intermittently sad, stressed, and emotional, and often all three at once, when visiting the facility. That was a relief to me, to know I was not alone in feeling emotional during my visits. Sandra also related to me that she had made several calls to the facility to see if her mother was being fed, because she kept getting calls from her mother saying "They are trying to starve me here.

They don't feed me." Luckily for Sandra, she wasn't labeled as "suspicious."

Lessons Learned

Try your best not to act out of pure emotion. Watching the mental and/or physical decline of a loved one is an emotionally difficult experience, but when we are reactionary and quick to jump to conclusions as a result of our emotional state, we generally do not handle situations as well as we might with a clear head.

If you or a loved one has legitimate concerns about the care or policies of a facility, make a list and an appointment to calmly discuss your concerns and/or questions. Guard against coming across as suspicious and accusatory, as it makes it more difficult for all parties involved (especially YOU).

TWENTY
Alternate Housing

I could not shake the growing desire to move my parents to a different facility. I learned of a private home called "Aspen Place" that had been transformed into a facility for the elderly and happened to have openings for two people, one man and one woman. After visiting with the nurse/administrator of this home on the telephone and feeling good about its possibilities, I visited and thought that this home would be a wonderful improvement for my parents. My dad would be able to "escape" the lock-down unit at Cedar Grove, and Mom wouldn't have to walk so far to see him; in fact, she'd hardly have to walk at all. A former private home, 8-10 residents now lived at Aspen Place, which was staffed 24 hours a day. It reminded me of a house that a group of diverse college students might share. One of the caregivers cooked all the meals, and the residents ate around a large oval table in the dining room.

Mom and Dad would stay in separate rooms, each with a roommate, which would definitely be a change. Mom was a very private person, so I wasn't sure how having a roommate would be received. One of the most positive parts for me, personally, was that the house was less than a five-minute drive from my home, compared with across town to the current facility. Being acutely anxious about choosing the "right" place for my parents, I decided to do a little homework this time, and asked for references. I called the relatives of three of the current residents to see how they liked the setup. All gave the home, the caregivers, and the administrator glowing reviews.

The next step was to take Mom for a visit and a meal, so she might see for herself what an improvement a move to this house could be for her and Dad. So confident was I of the logic of this choice that I had a "notification of move" letter typed and ready to deliver to the current facility administrator when I returned Mom to Cedar Grove, after what I was sure would be a successful visit. A month's notice before moving was required by Cedar Grove, and I didn't want to waste a single day.

The moment Mom and I walked in the door at Aspen Place, I realized we were in trouble. We were greeted by an overly excited, yapping dog scampering underfoot, a squawking bird fluttering around a small cage, and a mass of people all crowding into the dining room to find a seat for lunch. It was nothing short of chaotic. This was completely different from my prior mid-afternoon visit when all was serene. I could sense my mother's disdain before we'd even been in the house for five minutes. Mom and I were invited to sit down at the dining table with the other residents. The cook served tacos, and I noticed that Mom barely touched hers. It was messy to eat, and she wasn't even trying. This was not looking good. I over-compensated by talking non-stop, "interviewing" all the other women at the table (it was a table of all women this day), hoping that one of these women might spark Mom's interest and draw her into the conversation. Mom sat with her head down, and I sadly realized the lump in the pit of my stomach was not from over-eating.

Not willing to admit defeat after the seemingly unsuccessful lunch, I took her on a tour of the home. I showed her the small chair-like elevator she could ride up and down the stairs to the lower level. I introduced her to the woman who would be her prospective roommate, and toured the bedroom she would live in. I also showed her the bedroom Dad would live in, which was across the hall from her. Mom was polite, but distant and disengaged the entire time.

The Aspen Place nurse/administrator caught up with us after we toured the bedrooms on the lower level and showed us the bathroom the women shared and mentioned something about mandatory weekly checks for UTI's. Maybe it was the administrator's tone of voice or her delivery, but I once again thought of the movie version of *One Flew Over the Cuckoo's Nest*. This nurse conjured up thoughts of Nurse Ratched, and it was a slightly uncomfortable feeling that made me wonder if, in my zeal for finding new lodging for my parents, my intuition about this home had somehow misfired.

A bit later, as Mom and I sat alone on the couch in the lower level common room, Mom informed me, "Okay, Vicki, I'm ready to leave." I started backpedaling and encouraging her, "Mom, don't you like the cozy feeling in this house? Wouldn't it be great to be so close to Dad and not have so far to walk every day? This will be like moving into a house with a few roommates, plus it's so close to my house!" As I continued to list positive aspects of moving, inside it felt like I was sinking in quicksand as Mom pulled further and further into herself. She was done listening to me. Using a deep and overly dramatic voice, she looked me square in the eye and delivered her final comment on the whole idea: "It will kill me if you make us move here." Well, what could I say to that? I felt it important to give her some control over the decision, even though the experts I'd spoken with regarding the possibility of moving them (including her doctor and the nurse/administrator of Aspen Place) told me that circumstances had probably reached a point where I needed to seize control and do what I thought was best for my parents. At this particular time, I wasn't ready to take charge and intervene, so I instead demurred to my mother's wishes and dropped the whole plan. It was discouraging because of the positive reviews I'd received, and despite the nurse/administrator's protocol about checks for UTIs, I was so certain that this time I had made a better choice.

It had seemed like such a good idea in the beginning, but Mom's reticence, combined with my slight unease about "Nurse Ratched" ultimately helped me to forget the proposal. A year later as I was driving by Aspen Place, I noticed a "for sale" sign; upon inquiry, I learned that the facility had closed because the nurse/administrator hadn't been able to keep it running due to a lack of qualified caregivers. My thoughts returned to that uncomfortable feeling I'd felt around her, and I wondered if her personality had anything to do with the closure. In the end, I realized it was fortunate that I had not moved my parents there.

Lessons Learned

Carefully weigh the consequences of moving a loved one to a new facility. Will the move ultimately be beneficial, even though your loved one may not agree? Revisit your original parameters for selecting a facility to be sure you stay focused on those when looking at new facilities.

TWENTY-ONE
The Psychiatrist

After living at Cedar Grove for two years, Mom began seeing a psychiatrist for escalating paranoia and depression. Upon visiting my mother in her apartment and doing an assessment, Dr. Nielson, the psychiatrist, was amazed that my mother was still living on her own, and told me it was only because I "enabled" it; without me keeping such a close eye on Mom's needs, Dr. Nielson was convinced Mom would not be able to live on her own. Languishing in my own state of denial, I brushed this assessment aside.

In all honesty, when I felt most overwhelmed as the primary family caregiver, I sometimes selfishly fantasized about moving them back to Nelson City, if only to escape the daily anxiety and stress associated with them living nearby. Then I would remember the very institutionalized feel in the Nelson City facility—the cold, linoleum floors, standard-issue hospital beds, hospital-like cafeteria food, and the tiny "living" area for residents to sit and watch television. I found it to be a depressing place, and not somewhere I visualized my mother living with any quality of life. Even so, I second guessed myself and questioned my decision to move them to Coulson, wondering if it would have been better for them to remain in their hometown. It would have obviously been impossible for me to be as involved and available. Even though they both still repeatedly asked to go home, and my father continually asked where the car was, I realized that moving them closer to me had been the correct choice. Interestingly, one thing that clearly persisted for my father amidst all his other confusion was that he wasn't in his hometown. He may not have known where he was, but he knew it wasn't "home."

My motivation to help my mother stay in her apartment on her "own" for as long as possible was fueled in part by my ongoing guilt for having moved them to Coulson. My mother had always loved being in control, so by enabling her to stay in her own apartment, I could give her (and perhaps myself) the illusion that she was still somewhat in control of her daily life. As Alzheimer's disease continued to eat away at her brain, I saw how it scared her to lose more and more control. My mother had so much more awareness than my father of what was happening, and fought it tooth and nail.

This gives me pause for thought, as the Alzheimer's medication she took seemed to be a double-edged sword. On the one hand, she lived on her own longer, but on the other hand, her astute awareness of what she was losing as compared to my father, who was not taking any medication for Alzheimer's, created anguish for her. My dad was such a complacent man, who took life in stride without complaint. Was it worthwhile for Mom to take this medication and did it *really* improve her quality of life, or did the medication increase her awareness enough that it made letting go more painful? Today this is a moot point, but worth taking into consideration when deciding about Alzheimer's medications.

Why didn't Dad take the medication? I believe we thought his dementia and his age were far enough advanced that medication would be of little use for him. It seemed like a good idea for Mom to take the medication because, at the time, she was functioning at a much higher level than my dad. Is it better to administer Alzheimer's medication or not? What is the "right" choice? Did my mother's anguish, and my father's complacency, result from their distinct personality types, and have nothing to do with Alzheimer's medications? As caregivers, I believe that all we can do is exercise our best judgment in each given situation, and not agonize over the decision later, as I did.

Lessons Learned

Remember that you are doing the best you can with the information at hand. Situations can change in an instant, and it will be necessary to adjust the course of care accordingly, maybe even several times. Be open to these fluctuations, and try your best to adjust to the changing situation, whether that means changing your loved one's facility, doctor, medication, financial arrangements, etc. Do not hesitate to reach out for help from someone who has the expertise and knowledge to assist you.

TWENTY-TWO
Misadventures

Lionel and I went on a multi-day organized cycling trip across southern Utah in June of 2007. Because of sporadic phone service, I was unable to call each day to check in with Mom. When I eventually called mid-week, my mother was quick to inform, "Oh, Vicki. Something is wrong with me! There is this black liquid coming out of me! I don't know what to do. It happens every night after supper." And then she tacked on, "Something is wrong with your Dad, too."

"Oh dear, that sounds awful." I assumed she had a gastrointestinal bug, causing diarrhea. "I'm so sorry to hear this. Do you want me to call the staff nurse to check on you?"

"Oh no, there's nothing she could do." I let that go, thinking I would monitor it by calling the facility and visiting with the staff nurse anyway.

"Mom, what's wrong with Dad?" She couldn't exactly tell me what it was. We played our usual "20 Questions" as I tried to guess what she was trying to say, and she endeavored to find the appropriate words to convey her thoughts. Her broken thought processes and waning ability to retrieve words were frustrating to us both. Sometimes I could figure it out, and sometimes I couldn't. This time I couldn't.

The facility knew I was out of town, and knew to call me if there was an emergency, but I had received no calls or messages from them. When she repeated the same story the next day, I decided to call The Cottage to find out if Dad was ill. I learned he had developed an infected boil in his armpit, but that it wasn't classified as an emergency situation.

Our cycling tour ended that day, and we drove home the next day. I assured the facility nurse that we would take care of the boil situation upon our arrival. Once back in Coulson, our first stop was the Cedar Grove Alzheimer's Cottage, where Lionel addressed my dad's boil. Upon examination, he determined the boil had already drained, and was starting to diminish. My husband discussed the care plan with the staff, to keep an eye on the healing boil. Once the situation with my dad was under control, and we'd spent some time visiting with both Mom and Dad, Lionel and I returned to our house in the late afternoon to begin unpacking. We thought all would be well, until about 9 p.m. that evening when our telephone rang. It was Mom, who spoke in a hushed voice, "Vicki, I had a little accident on the way to the toilet. Could you come over?" I rushed to her apartment to see she had, shall we say, released loose fecal matter in many locations, leaving a trail between her bed and the bathroom.

I have an undying admiration for caregivers in these facilities. Because of her sense of propriety, and the fact my mother lived "independently," she didn't call anyone in the facility for help, and it was very humiliating for her to even have to call me. As not to upset her further, I didn't make a big deal out of it—I simply cleaned the carpet and floor of her apartment. I put all the soiled towels, sheets, and bedclothes in a big pile to take home and wash, helped her put on fresh pajamas, put clean sheets on her bed, and tucked her in.

She looked so tiny and fragile laying there when I kissed her good night, and moments like this struck me how thoroughly lonely and sad she seemed. What did she have to look forward to tomorrow or next week? Struggling to dress herself each morning, which she told me took nearly an hour (she was too proud to ask for help), eating breakfast, spending time with Dad, eating her noontime dinner, spending more time with Dad, eating supper, and then going to her apartment and preparing for bed alone? She still had the ability to watch a bit of TV, but said the programs were so awful that it was not worth turning on (I agreed with her about that). She insisted that television programs in Nelson City were much more interesting, even though Nelson City aired the same programming as Coulson. She could no longer write, but she could still read, although her comprehension was fading, day-by-day, month-by-month. Is this how it ends? Does it have to be so?

I yearned to find something for her that would help occupy part of her day. She appeared to spend most of the time worrying about money and my father, and scratching her body in a very nervous manner. She continued to be unhappy, lonely, and depressed. On Mom's most recent visit, Dr. Nielson increased the dose of her antidepressant. It takes some time for the increased medication to take effect, however, and it had yet to make much of a difference.

There are times when I simply don't understand life. Driving home that night after tucking Mom into bed, I gave in to the overwhelming feelings of helplessness and wept, letting the unabated tears stream down my face. I wept for my mother and her losses; I wept for all elderly people who feel like there is nothing to do all day, with nothing to look forward to. I selfishly cried for myself, for the loss of the parents I once knew, and the fear that I may end up in the same place years from now. I have often told friends, "Well, when I am old, I may lose the ability to be as active as I now am, but at least I can enjoy my abundant memories." I used to say that, but with my genetics, sadly, I dare not say that now.

Lesson Learned

If you are out of town and there is any doubt or question about the well-being of your loved one, do not wait for the facility to call you; call them.

TWENTY-THREE
Social Security Matters

Since statements from government agencies were not bills to be paid, I did not worry too much if Mom threw some away. I admit I had procrastinated on changing the mailing address to mine because of the paperwork involved. However, because of the lingering possibility that she might "accidentally" toss out mail that was important, I eventually had to go through the process of becoming the representative payee for Social Security. This was the only way I could receive their insurance, Medicare and Social Security statements at my home address. When one becomes a representative payee, the Social Security Administration sends a letter to the payee explaining his or her government mail will now be sent to his or her representative payee, which in my parents' case was me. This is done in order to protect the payee from identity theft and to verify the payee is in agreement with the change. For people that have paranoia, understanding a letter stating that their social security checks will now be going to another family member can be hard to comprehend, especially if that person already makes a habit of accusing said family member of stealing their money. It's not hard to imagine what happened when Mom read *that* letter.

"Hello?"

"Vicki?"

"Oh, hi Mom. How are you today?"

"Not. Very. Good," she said slowly and emphatically. "My daughter is stealing my money," she continued in a low-pitched, frosty voice.

I sighed and thought to myself, *do we have to go here yet again? And, what is she talking about? It must be serious because she's back to talking about me in the third person.*

I managed to muster a confused, yet innocent, "Mom, please tell me what you're talking about."

"After all we've done for you, how could you do this?" The volume of her shrill-sounding voice escalated with each subsequent word.

"Mom, please tell me what you're talking about," I pleaded with her, carefully repeating my question using the same words, so as not to further confuse her.

"I have the letter in my hand right now, and it says you're stealing our Social Security money."

I realized she must be referring to some letter she received from the Social Security Administration, but I could not imagine what the letter said that would cause such a reaction from her.

"Mom, this is some sort of mix-up. I'm not taking your Social Security money! It will still be automatically deposited into your account each month, the same as always."

"That's not what this letter says."

"Mom, I would never steal your money! Listen, I'm on my way to see you right now, and we'll get this straightened out, I promise."

"Don't bother to come. You're fired!" she screamed into my ear. And in a very dramatic voice, she added, "Stay away." She then slammed down the receiver.

It was as if I could physically feel the impact of the crashing receiver reverberating in my head. I took a few deep breaths, grabbed my car keys, and ran out the back door.

When I arrived at her apartment, the door was left slightly ajar. *So, even though she told me to stay away, she knew*

I'd come. When I entered, however, I didn't find her waiting for me. In glancing around the apartment I noticed her bedroom door was shut, and realized she was probably hiding in there. I found the Social Security letter on her card table. I skimmed the text of the letter and realized why she was so upset.

" *... we are writing to tell you that we have information that shows you need help managing your money and meeting your needs. Because of this information, we plan to send your Social Security benefits to Vicki Tapia. We will call this PERSON your representative payee ...* "

The letter explained that my parents could appeal the decision, or hire a lawyer to help them if they disagreed with the decision to appoint me as representative payee. It became clear why I had subconsciously procrastinated this address change.

I walked to her bedroom door and knocked, gently asking her to come out so I could explain the letter to her. Begrudgingly she acquiesced, and we sat down to discuss the text of the letter. We called the Social Security Office, and waited on hold for one hour so that their representative could also explain to Mom what the letter meant (echoing my earlier explanation). While Mom acted like she understood the lengthy explanations, I'm not sure the government worker or I ever really convinced her that her Social Security benefit check would continue to be deposited into her checking account, just as it had always been. I left her apartment that day wishing I could write a letter to the person in charge of drafting Social Security letters, and tell them what I thought of their letters.

Unfortunately, it seemed the things that I wished Mom would forget were the very things that obsessively imbedded themselves into her failing memory. This was neither the first nor the last time that she tried to "fire" me. There would be more moments when I wished I really *could* have been "fired," or at least quit!

Over time I developed a thicker skin—an act of self-preservation. I learned how to emotionally distance myself from her wild ranting and crazy accusations. I consoled myself with the realization that this person was no longer the mother I knew, but some sad, demented woman who did not understand what she was saying or doing.

On a side note, in becoming the representative payee for my parents, I discovered that the clerk who input the Social Security information for my father when he retired in 1974 had spelled Dad's last name incorrectly. It takes little imagination to understand the added stress I experienced straightening out *this* mess. No one wants to know what it was like dealing with the government to fix an error that was 23 years old.

Lessons Learned

Give short explanations, and allow your loved one an abundance of time to comprehend what you have said. Always repeat sentences using the same words; when you repeat a sentence using different words it easily confuses them.

If you elect to become representative payee, be forewarned that your loved one will be receiving a letter detailing the change. Be prepared for potential irrational accusations. Consider making a call to the Social Security office after the letter arrives to let their representative explain it to your loved one.

TWENTY-FOUR
The Curious Occurrence of the Comet Cleanser

Mom's shoes had developed a pervasive stench. There was no other way to describe it. In hindsight, I realize it may have been related to the fact that she continuously wore the same pair of leg-support knee-highs. I was somehow deluded into thinking she washed them occasionally. Now I realize she probably did not. I could have been more proactive about washing them myself, but she always wore them, and did not want an additional pair as she felt the cost was too expensive. It would have been an excellent idea if I had bought her a second pair anyway, and helped her change them each week, and then washed the pair she had been wearing. *Why, oh why, didn't I think of that?* It now seems like a no-brainer. Perhaps I was still maneuvering through various and changing forms of denial. In any case, the next best thing was a bottle of foot odor remover. I showed her how to sprinkle some of the white powder in her shoes each morning. This really helped with the odor.

One day, several weeks later, I visited her and noticed the yellow plastic bottle of Comet cleanser I had brought to clean her sink and toilet sitting on her nightstand in her bedroom. I found this a little odd, so I asked her, "Mom, why is the Comet cleanser on your bedroom nightstand shelf?"

She replied, "Well, I am sprinkling it in my shoes every morning, just like you told me to!"

She tried so hard to follow directions. My heart went out to her for trying. Well, at least her shoes were very clean inside, and the bottoms of her feet sparkling! I replaced the *appropriate* bottle of foot odor remover by her bedside, and brought the Comet cleanser home with me. I am reminded of her every time I clean our toilets!

My mother did not take kindly to what she considered "interference" with her housekeeping. Because she had always been such an immaculate housekeeper, walking into her apartment and seeing her bathroom sink caked with grime and an ever-growing brown ring around the toilet bowl was one more reminder that her brain function was deteriorating. Whenever I thought I could carefully, yet unobtrusively, clean the sink or toilet without her noticing I seized the opportunity. However, I sensed that change loomed on the horizon.

Lessons Learned

Have more awareness than I did, and buy an extra pair of support hose! Wash the extra pair in the sink whenever you visit.

Assisted-living facilities typically have a cleaning service, but Mom refused to let them come into her apartment. Should this be the case for you, and hygiene/sanitary living conditions become an issue, consider arriving while the loved one is otherwise occupied (on a bus ride or in the dining room eating, for example), clean the grime off the sink and toilet, and change the towels and sheets while he or she is away. It is unlikely to even be noticed, but you will have the peace of mind knowing the living space is clean. Bring cleaning supplies with you when you visit and remove them when you leave.

TWENTY-FIVE
Struggles

The three of us struggled through the third summer at Cedar Grove. My mother's behavior was often angry as well as paranoid, and usually directed towards me. Her psychiatrist, Dr. Nielson, approached me and told me I was showing signs of "burnout," and should seriously consider moving my parents somewhere else, where there was more supervision for Mom and a shorter distance for her to walk to visit my father, because of her faltering mobility. The lock-down Cottage where my dad currently resided didn't seem appropriate for Mom, plus the cost of living at this facility was climbing at a pace that my parents were not going to be able to sustain indefinitely.

Dr. Nielson gave me the names of a couple of facilities with which she was familiar, and strongly encouraged me to visit them. I put the note on my desk, and each day it stared back at me, as if imploring me to act. I almost threw it away several times because I reasoned that it would be too difficult to move my parents. *Difficult for whom? Me? The two of them?* Every time I thought of moving them, it gave me a sense of dread and foreboding. One of my major concerns was how difficult such a change might be for them. I wasn't sure I could cope with the moving process, let alone Mom's reaction, which was sure to be stormy. In my mind, I kept re-living the catastrophe of my mother's visit to Aspen Place. That little note did not give up, however, and gazed back at me from its seemingly secure position on my desk. After several weeks of visual sparring with the note, I relented and thought, "Well, it wouldn't hurt to look."

One day I impulsively picked up this note with the phone numbers, contemplated them for a minute, and called the first facility on the list. It happened to be right across the street from Cedar Grove. I liked what I heard on the phone and drove over to see it that very afternoon. I was excited by what I observed. My parents could be in rooms next door to each other. The downside, apart from the move itself, was Mom's living space. She would no longer have her own apartment—only a bedroom with a half-bath, something I knew she would not easily accept.

It was mid-summer, and my older daughter, Megan, was home visiting. One afternoon we visited my parents, and asked them to take a walk with us. The two of us strolled with Mom, as we pushed Dad in his wheelchair across the street to tour this other facility. Dad's reaction was his usual, non-committal "whatever" self. Mom, on the other hand, seemed to warm to the idea of being in a room right next door to Dad, and not having to walk so far to see him.

Tendercare Cottages had a lovely set-up; all the bedrooms, each with a half-bath, hugged the perimeter of the rectangular building, with three rooms opening onto the large, sunny common area with a living room, dining room, and kitchen, where the staff prepared the meals. The two rooms currently available happened to be those opening onto that common area. The facility was a smaller cottage-style with only 16 residents (no shared rooms), compared with more than 100 at Cedar Grove. This would definitely be a more intimate setting and my mother could have the closer supervision that her psychiatrist recommended. Each bedroom had a large window overlooking a grassy area behind the building, as well as a windowed door that opened onto a sidewalk circling the building. Beyond the small lawn outside the two available rooms was a tall white fence, which bordered the perimeter of the complex along a busy street. The fence effectively blocked out the sound of traffic and kept residents from wandering away, which would eventually prove beneficial for my father's safety.

The caregivers would be in charge of dispensing Mom's medications, so we would know for sure she was taking them at the right time and in the right amount. I had removed her osteoporosis medication altogether at this point, as it appeared she was taking a pill whenever she thought about it despite the clearly marked calendar I'd set up to assist her. Recently when organizing her pills, I found only two remaining osteoporosis pills when there should have been six. Because no one was there to see that she took the pill on the appointed day when she awakened, who knew what was happening? It gave me a sense of relief to know that at Tendercare Cottages, a caregiver would dispense her medications; it was one less thing for me to obsess about.

At Tendercare Cottages, I had assurance that her bed sheets and towels would be changed regularly, and someone was always nearby if she needed help. She was so isolated in her apartment at Cedar Grove that I felt compelled to call every evening to be sure she was all right. I knew she was having trouble doing her laundry when she called me one night and asked, "How do you make the machine work?"

"What machine, Mom?" I asked her.

"You know," as she struggled for the right words.

"Um, your television?" No response. "Clock? Microwave? Answering machine?" I started guessing, naming all the machines I could think of until I finally hit the right one: "Your washing machine?"

"Yes!"

I then attempted to describe which button to push. At the end of this telephone conversation, I was fairly certain we had not communicated clearly, and I doubted she would be washing any clothes that evening.

Prior to her washing machine SOS call, I had begun to notice that her clothing wasn't completely clean much of the time, and I suspected she wasn't washing her sheets and towels very often either, if at all. Whenever I tactfully suggested that I might be able to help her change her bedding because I knew it was "difficult with the arthritis," she was quite indignant and insistent that she could do it herself. Injuring herself in the process of making her bed, either by tripping or becoming tangled in bed sheets was a real possibility. I constantly walked the fine line between respecting her and keeping her safe. The two were often in direct opposition to one another. Some battles were worth fighting, and some were not. I decided the dirty-clothes battle was probably not worth fighting at that moment, and to my dismay, her clothing remained somewhat rumpled and stained.

As we stood in this new facility that hot summer afternoon, I felt amazement that Mom did not begin her mantra of "no, no, no" in response to the idea of moving. Taking advantage of her agreeable mood, I promptly wrote out the deposit check for their rooms on the spot. The wheels had finally been set in motion. A huge wave of relief immediately washed over me.

I hadn't been home more than a couple of hours when Mom called to say, "I've talked it over with your father, and we've decided we don't want to move. We're happy where we are, so you can just forget it!" Her words were uncharacteristically clear and succinct.

I couldn't say, "Well, sorry, you don't get to vote," so I simply listened, and even attempted to reason with her a bit, knowing all the while it was futile. There was little chance my dad had *actually* said he didn't want to move. I can imagine the conversation:

Mom would have said something like, "You don't want to move, do you?"

My ever-compliant dad might have replied, "No," probably not even fully comprehending the question.

Thus ensued a battle of wills, tears, temper tantrums, demands, and suicidal threats (these last three being my mother's reactions).

"If you make me move, I will kill myself. I'm going to just go jump into the river." Or, "Please bring my papers and money to me; I have no further need of you. The girls here will help me."

I know that this was part dementia, and part loss of control over life. Most of us control our own lives—we decide when to get up, when to go to bed, what and how much to eat, what to wear, and how to spend our days. Relinquishing control over daily life would be difficult for anyone, but for my mother, with her controlling personality, it was even more so.

Mom began calling my house many times a day, alternately sobbing and begging me not to move them, and then yelling at the top of her voice that they weren't going to move under any circumstance. I stopped talking about it, and I think she thought she had "won," and that I'd given up on moving them because life resumed some sort of normalcy for a few brief days.

During this period of calm, much like the eye of a storm, I visited her one afternoon, and we sat together on her bed. She watched me sew errant buttons back onto several of her blouses. In my memory, this was our last conversation that had a sense of normalcy. It was as if she was magically "herself" again for a brief period of time. We chatted amicably, and while I can't remember the details of the conversation, I vividly remember thinking this is what it was like when Mom was Mom. This afternoon remains an often-savored treasure stored in my memory. I did not want that afternoon together on her bed to come to an end, as if I knew I'd been granted this one last time to connect with the mother I remembered.

The truce was short-lived. Soon she started to call me at home to bargain. "If you'll let us stay here, I'll move into The Cottage with your dad." Although that might have been a possibility, the new facility was much more in line with what both of them needed in a facility, including not being locked down with the severely demented individuals at Cedar Grove. Another more practical reason to move them was the fact that the price was $1,200 less a month. When spending nearly $7,000 a month for two was reduced to $5,800 a month, along with better surroundings, it became easy to make a decision. My dilemma was how to explain that to Mom with her dementia. Cedar Grove decided to complicate things a bit by offering to reduce their price to match the $5,800 a month for a period of one year. I wasn't tempted and didn't tell Mom of that offer.

In retrospect, it's evident that I eliminated emotion from my decision, and instead focused on logic and intellect in making the choice to move them to a different facility. I distanced myself from my mother's agony in my attempt to keep her safe (*and to protect myself, as well?*). I could not have predicted how excruciating this move would ultimately prove for her. She was crying out in pain once again at the loss of what had become comfortable and familiar to her. I was the villain taking away everything she knew and understood. I don't know how I could have made this less painful for her, but here I was again, inflicting my decisions upon her against her will; yet, I made this decision with my parents' best interests at heart. With her limited cognition, she was unable to understand this, and in the midst of it, I was unable to find the right approach to ease the transition. I regret this, because I don't feel she ever recovered from this last move, but only declined at a quicker pace. *Because I forced the move, am I responsible for hastening her decline?* I asked myself repeatedly.

Our contract with Cedar Grove stipulated a mandatory one-month notice before moving. Because Mom was having such a difficult time and acting out with public displays of sobbing and wailing, the administrator at Cedar Grove called and told me "We'll waive the month moving notice if you're able to move your parents sooner. It's difficult to watch your mother's torment and agony, and we don't wish to prolong it longer than necessary." All I *heard* was "Get her the *hell* out of here; the sooner, the better." I can't imagine that her public wailing was good for business, either. We pushed the moving day forward by two weeks.

Lessons Learned

Burnout is very real. Pay attention when someone tells you that you are showing signs of it, and take appropriate action before it overtakes you. Carefully pick your battles, because not all battles are worth the tears and anguish they often cause. In Mom's case, it might have been easier if I'd remained calm and only listened and made no attempt to reason with her. These are the times when it's necessary to remove all emotion and act with logic and in the best interests of the person for whom you are caring. Keep in mind your own mental health.

According to the experts, signs of caregiver burnout include:

* Withdrawal from friends, family, or other loved ones

* Losing interest in outside activities previously enjoyed
* Feelings of irritability, hopelessness, or helplessness
* Changes in sleep patterns
* Becoming ill more often
* Wanting to hurt either yourself or the person you are caring for
* Exhaustion, both physical and mental

TWENTY-SIX
Moving Day...Take Two

Moving day approached. The calls from my demented mother increased in their intensity, to the point of me often ignoring the phone when it rang. Once, I handed the phone to Lionel, and upon placing the receiver to his ear he heard a feeble, "Please, please can you help me?"

He replied in his typically calm voice, "How can I help you?"

She said, "You can bring all my money and papers to me, and tell your wife to get out of my life."

He listened to her, and gave her the opportunity to calm down, and then assured her that he'd do his best to help her. That seemed to placate her for the time being, and the call ended shortly thereafter.

I'm surprised that she even remembered I was his wife, or who he was. In some conversations, I was still attempting to reason with her, which I forgot was a futile idea. For example, I asked her, "Mom, who will take care of all the day-to-day paperwork and appointments if you fire me?" She answered in a nasty voice, "Oh, don't you worry about that, Miss Smarty Pants. I've already asked the girls here, and they told me they would do everything I need done. So, you can just pack up and bring me all my papers. I don't want to see you again."

"Okay, Mom, whatever you say," I lied to her, as I had no intention of complying with this demand. Amazingly, once in a while her powers of speech returned with a vengeance. It is difficult when the child has to become the parent. Mom was now acting like a 15-year-old teenager with unrealistic ideas, along with the sullenness often characterizing that age group.

It was at this time that I called and literally begged my brother to come to Coulson, and help me get through the move.

"Would you consider flying here to spend a few days? I really, *really* need your support. Mom is falling apart over this whole move, and I think I may fall apart with her!"

He said jokingly, "We must have a bad connection on the phone line, because I can't hear what you are saying."

"This is not *funny*," I said curtly, "and I am *not* in the mood to joke about it."

In the background, I heard his wife, Rhoda, saying, "She wants you to buy a plane ticket and go out there? Well, *that* would be a waste of money."

I was amazed and angered by this attitude. *They don't understand what this is like*, I thought to myself.

He went on, "Rhoda and I prefer to remember Mom and Dad the way they were."

The way they were? I can't believe I am having this conversation, I thought to myself and responded, bitterly, "What was I thinking?"

Seemingly oblivious to my sarcasm, he offered, "How about if we help pay for the moving expenses?"

"It isn't financial support I am looking for," I countered, "it's *emotional* support that I so desperately need."

It was obvious to me that my statements were falling upon deaf ears, and the conversation ended shortly. It saddened me that I was unable to communicate to my only sibling how desperate I felt. It was sadder still that he couldn't give the loving support only a sibling could provide in a situation such as this. I am, however, forever grateful and thankful to have the undying support of my husband throughout this journey. Oddly enough, reflecting on this time and my interactions with my brother gives me an idea of how my mother must have been feeling, even in her demented state. I wasn't listening to her plead with me not to move her and Dad, and my brother wasn't listening to me begging him to come and help me get through the move. It's all relative, is it not?

Four days before the scheduled move, Aunt Lydia, my dad's sister-in-law, passed away in our hometown of Nelson City. The funeral was unfortunately scheduled for our moving day, July 31. The thought of rearranging the moving date in order to attend her funeral was far too overwhelming to contemplate, so my understanding husband drove with me two hours late in the afternoon the day before the funeral/moving day to attend my aunt's wake. Stressful though it was, I know it was the right decision to see my cousins and honor my aunt in this way.

The morning after the wake, Lionel and I were up early to drive home and face the big moving day. We had an elaborate plan laid out and, happily, it actually worked! One of the caregivers from Cedar Grove wheeled my father over to Tendercare Cottages mid-morning, and then returned for Mom, who was in her apartment. The caregiver offered to drive my mother over, but she angrily said she would, "walk, thank you very much." It was probably a good idea they walked, because the caregiver later commented to me, "It occurred to me that I might never have been able to pry your mother out of my car, had I driven."

Mom was furious with my dad, whom she believed had betrayed her, when she walked through the door and she saw him sitting in the common room of the new facility. I was told her eyes were blazing (practically throwing sparks, to be precise) as she demanded to know why he had "agreed to the move." He didn't really seem to have any clue what was going on, and gently stared back at her without saying anything. This was typical for him; his lack of reaction was simply more maddening to my mother.

Knowing my presence would undoubtedly upset Mom, I stationed myself at Cedar Grove to pack up their belongings after they left. Lionel and two of the work crew from Tendercare Cottages moved all the boxes and furniture. My job was to sort, pack, toss, and tidy up. Dad's room was first. I looked around his room, realizing there wasn't much for me to pack, only what was left of his clothing and a few odds and ends, like his clock and recently repaired shaver. There were two paintings from their home in Nelson City that I'd rehang in his new room, which would give some continuity in the midst of change. I maintained a business-like attitude, because if I didn't, I thought I might cry realizing how little my Dad had left of his former, full life.

Once his room was cleared and his belongings were transported to Tendercare Cottages, I moved on to Mom's apartment, which would be much more time-consuming. Her plates, bowls, utensils, and other kitchenware would find a temporary home in my attic. Except for her recliner and bedroom set, the rest of her furniture would be delivered to a used furniture/consignment store. Clothes, knick-knacks, wall art, and her toiletries went into boxes for the trip across the street to their new home at Tendercare Cottages.

On one of Lionel's deliveries of their belongings, my mother, fussing and fuming on the couch in the common area of Tendercare Cottages, informed him, "Tell your wife she need not visit us here." He told her he would pass along the message. It was a relief for me to spout out the word, "fine," to him when he gave me the news. I was definitely ready for a break, and felt relieved I wouldn't have to talk to her. Realistically, I knew that it wouldn't last.

I continued to practice distancing myself from her constant barrage in the name of self-preservation. I had come a long way from the grief and pain I once experienced whenever she verbally attacked me. I was now able to listen, compartmentalize, and realize that I need not take it personally; I reminded myself once again of my mantra that, "it's really not the mother I once knew who is speaking." It helped me considerably to learn how to be dispassionate about, and divorce myself from, emotional entanglement with this demented woman. This is not to say that I didn't hug, kiss, and love her when I was with her, but when she went on her tirades, I no longer found myself buying into it, which in the past caused me to fall apart with her.

Mom's silence lasted a mere 48 hours before I received a phone call. I confess, I groaned, as I had hoped for a longer respite! Her first question was, "Why are you ignoring us?" I was out to visit that very afternoon and perceived they were settling in nicely. I experienced a bit of whiplash when Mom commented on how wonderful it was at this facility, how kind the caregivers were, how delicious the food tasted, and how terrific it was to be so close to Dad. She was still clearly upset that I made them move, however, and told me I was "sneaky." So be it. Mission accomplished. She seemed to be making the best of it.

Lessons Learned

There are resources available for maneuvering through elder care with siblings. This is an area I didn't realize existed at the time I was in the midst of it, and in retrospect, wish I had thought to investigate. One of the suggestions I particularly liked was to set aside a time every week to discuss how things were going for Mom and Dad. I wonder if that might have helped the communication between my brother and me.

For more information:

Mom Always Liked You Best: A Guide for Resolving Family Feuds, Inheritance Battles, & Eldercare Crises by Arline Kardasis et al.

They're Your Parents, Too! How Siblings Can Survive Their Parents' Aging Without Driving Each Other Crazy by Francine Russo

A Bittersweet Season: Caring for Our Aging Parents—And Ourselves by Jane Gross

TWENTY-SEVEN
The Honeymoon Is Over

For several weeks, all was "peachy," and I prayed it would last, but deep down I had an uneasy feeling it was only a temporary state of affairs. Each day, Mom told me how much she liked the new facility, and how tremendous the care was. I was savvy enough to realize we were in the honeymoon phase, but I soaked up every minute of it. Dad seemed completely content as well, and could easily wheel his way around the facility in his wheelchair. Dad's new room was more spacious than at Cedar Grove, so the facility brought in one of their recliners for him to use, placing it in front of the garden door, at the foot of his bed. Mom's bed was situated beneath her window next to her favorite turquoise recliner. I hoped that the familiarity of her own furniture made the room feel homey and the transition easier for her. So far, she hadn't made any disparaging remarks about downsizing from an apartment to a single room. As a final touch, Lionel and I had hung their pictures and paintings, dividing them between the two rooms.

There were activities at the facility that attracted Mom, including occasional entertainment, church, and sightseeing bus rides once a week, and lots of craft activities and games. I also asked the caregivers to include Mom in any little helpful chores, like folding towels or sorting silverware, because she liked to "stay busy." On occasion, they even gave her the broom to push down the halls, sweeping up miscellaneous crumbs and dust bunnies. She appeared to be adjusting splendidly, at least during daylight hours.

Although the days at Tendercare Cottages passed smoothly, the nights were another matter. After Mom had been there a few days, she turned up in the common room one evening about 9 p.m., stark naked. The night shift caregiver, Jody, quickly exclaimed, "Honey, you need to go back to your room and put your pajamas on."

Mom's response was less than poetic. "I'll do what I damn well please. You can't tell me what to do."

That was the beginning of an interesting evening for Mom and the caregiver, as after the "naked incident," she found Mom in someone else's room wearing a sweater belonging to that resident. Jody shooed Mom back into her room, only to thereafter find her in another resident's room trying to put on the man's pants. I was told Jody did manage to send Mom back into her own room for the rest of the night, where she eventually quieted down.

My mother had no memory of this the next day. I decided she must have been sleepwalking. When they called to report this incident to me, she also commented, "I don't know if you know this or not, but your mother sleeps naked. We were wondering if she's ever slept in pajamas?" I was speechless for a moment. *My mother was sleeping in the nude? This was definitely NOT my mother.*

"There should be several pairs of pajamas in her bureau. Could you please check to see if they're there? If they're gone, I'll bring her another pair."

"Sure, we'll check it out."

"Could you please help her into her pajamas at night?"

"Certainly!"

I hoped that would be the end of it, but little did I know, it was a new beginning.

This phone call reminded me of a similar incident regarding my dad when he was still at Cedar Grove. Mom and Dad hadn't lived there too many months at the time (could this be an adjustment thing?). My dad enjoyed getting out of his wheelchair and going to bed to relax for a while after the noon meal. One day, the caregivers were busy and forgot to lay him down, and he showed up in the dining room in his wheelchair, totally naked, in public no less! My quiet, conservative father, naked! Well, that was a shock, but I confess when I was informed of the incident, I had to chuckle and wonder in amazement how he managed to undress himself while confined to a wheelchair.

As I suspected, my mother's good humor was a temporary condition, and the "honeymoon" phase for her at the new facility was short-lived. After a few weeks, the complaining began again in earnest. "The food here is just stinking bad. These girls don't know how to cook worth a damn." Or, "They are so mean here. They yell at me!" "There is never anything to do here." Mom's ability to absorb and understand television programs or what she was reading had dramatically decreased. She continued to attempt to read the newspaper every morning to Dad, but in some ways it was like listening to a first grader learning to read by sounding out words. I don't know how much either of them got out of it, but it did help them to pass the morning. Mom was tenacious to the end. Even though it was a struggle to read, she did not give up. Listening to her made me anxious and became a lesson in patience as I struggled to withhold blurting out the word she was attempting to sound out.

I listened to her complaints and tried to follow up on them as much as possible. I also had to learn one more time that her perception of reality was not necessarily anyone else's. One day when she called, she lamented, "You know, those girls took my wig away from me! Can you imagine? So, now I can't wear it anymore." (Mom had occasionally begun wearing a wig years ago when they were popular because she thought that her hair was too thin and fine.) On my next visit, I found the wig shoved into the far corner on the top shelf in her closet. I questioned the caregivers because I had a hard time believing that *she* could have tossed it up there. They had no idea what I was talking about. They did relate that she'd worn her wig the day before and everyone had complimented her on it. It was only then that it began to dawn on me that my mother had somehow probably thrown the wig onto that top shelf, and was once again blaming her behavior on the caregivers.

It's hard to believe how slow I was to understand the behavior of an Alzheimer's patient, even though I had read the books, watched the documentaries, and had been caring for someone suffering from it for more than three years. My lack of clear understanding regarding some of the effects of this disease still surprises me. I wanted to believe what Mom told me, even though I suspected it was her committing the offensive act, and then blaming it on someone else; I wanted to think that she still had some sort of ability to report her life accurately. Why did I think this? *This was my mother, and she never lied to me. This was my mother, the person I had trusted my entire life. Of course I believed her!* I needed to reorient my thinking. There was also a sort of denial on my part, I suppose, hoping to have a conversation with my real mother, not this person who lived in another dimension. Over the past three plus years (and perhaps even longer), I felt I'd slowly peeled back the many layers of an onion, uncovering a deeper awareness of the many and varied behaviors of dementia.

Lessons Learned

Be creative in thinking of ways to make someone with dementia feel needed if they act restless like my mom. Ask the caregivers if they have any little "chores" your loved one can do to feel useful and help pass the time.

Be prepared for personality changes and erratic behavior.

I can't reiterate enough: remember to separate the person you once knew from the person currently before you. Remind yourself, yet again, to take her comments with a grain of salt, especially if they involve accusations toward others, and displaying out-of-the-ordinary behaviors.

TWENTY-EIGHT
Dad's Antics

By their third summer in Coulson, my father was in his third wheelchair; he had somehow managed to break off the leg/foot support piece, and the medical supply house found it necessary to supply a new chair when repairs didn't last. Given his track record with wheelchairs, I am thankful we decided to rent a wheelchair instead of buying.[5]

Because my father had a difficult time remembering that he couldn't walk, he often attempted to stand up from his wheelchair and walk on his own. This, of course, was incredibly dangerous, as he couldn't even stand unsupported on his own, let alone walk! Because of this risk, Cedar Grove had clipped a "tab alarm" to his shirt that buzzed loudly if the clip came off, as would be the case if he attempted to stand or move too far away from the alarm anchor, which was on the wheelchair itself. One day, after having lived in Cedar Grove for nearly a year, he attempted to stand up and walk, and despite our precautionary installation of the tab alarm to notify the caregivers, he had a hard fall. The resulting pain in his hip required a trip by ambulance to the hospital to rule out any broken bones.

Lionel, Dad, and I subsequently spent four hours in the hospital emergency department for x-rays and a CT-scan. Thankfully, nothing was broken, but he was sore for a while. Because of the ineffectiveness of the tab alarm alone,

[5]We had the option of buying or renting the wheelchair through Medicare. The best choice we made was to rent because of these breakdowns. If we had owned the wheelchair, we would have had to buy a new chair each time. The rent was covered by Medicare, so in the end, there was no cost to my parents. This also applied to Dad's hospital bed.

the doctor recommended a seat belt also be installed on his wheelchair to prevent further injuries. I do give him credit for his industriousness, because Dad quickly learned how to unbuckle the belt.

At times my dad's prostate cancer still caused him discomfort and an urgent, frequent need to urinate. After the move to Tendercare Cottages, he had a flare-up of his prostate cancer. He also had another new wheelchair, which hadn't had a seat belt installed yet. Because of this urgency to urinate, one day he attempted to stand up and fell, which meant a second trip to the hospital emergency department. This time he was not so fortunate, as x-rays showed a hairline fracture of his pelvis. Once back at Tendercare Cottages, pain medication provided only limited relief and my typically stoic Dad complained, so I knew he was uncomfortable. His appetite diminished, and his skin color had a slightly grey appearance. I began to wonder if we might lose him.

After a few weeks, the staff nurse at Tendercare Cottages suggested that his doctor see him, because she felt some physical therapy might help him sit more comfortably in his wheelchair and help with the healing process. Unfortunately, in the midst of this, my parents' primary care doctor moved out of state.

A new facility specializing in elder care had opened a practice only a few blocks from Tendercare Cottages. This seemed like an ideal time to transfer my parent's care to this facility, so I called to set up an appointment for Dad to see the new geriatric specialist. I was excited by the proximity of the medical facility, and felt that having an eldercare specialist would be an ideal arrangement for my parents. I requested my parents' massive medical files be sent from their former physician's office to this new medical facility, and completed all the necessary paperwork for the transfers. All that remained was to physically transfer Dad from Tendercare Cottages to the new medical facility on the day of his appointment. I was impressed by how quickly we were able to secure that appointment.

When the day of his appointment arrived, the administrator at Tendercare Cottages transported Dad in her SUV, rather than the facility bus, and met me in the parking lot of the medical facility. Once we had him unloaded and safely ensconced in his wheelchair, I wheeled him into the waiting area. The room had high ceilings, stone floors, and little warmth. There was no one else in the large room except for the receptionist. She was very welcoming and personable, which offset the coldness of the room, and I thought to myself, *so far, so good*. There was more paperwork to complete, so I sat down next to Dad to fill it out. Dad was obviously bored because when I looked up from the paperwork, I noticed that he had inserted his hand inside his pants to entertain himself. When he saw I was looking at him, he asked,

"What are we doing here?"

"We are waiting to see the doctor."

"Why?"

"Well, we hope to be able to get you some physical therapy to speed up your recovery from your last fall."

"Oh," was his uninterested reply, and he went back to more important matters. Knowing that one odd side effect of his Parkinson's medication was the urge to masturbate helped me to overlook incidents like this.

Eventually, we were directed to an exam room, where the nurse asked us questions regarding Dad's medical history. She was very thorough and kind. *I really like this nurse*, I thought, feeling more comfortable by the minute.

Shortly thereafter, the physician entered the room, and the whole tone changed. I had prepared myself to "like" this physician because she specialized in elder care, and I liked the proximity of her practice to Tendercare Cottages. I also liked how quickly the physician entered the room following the nurse's departure, as there is often a long wait between these two segments of a doctor's visit. A tall, thin, stern-looking woman met my gaze with piercing blue eyes. She had the frosty air of winter about her. Without saying a word to me, she immediately turned her attention to my dad.

"Well, Mr. Andersen, what can I do for you today?" she asked him.

My dad just looked at her blankly, and it was apparent he was not in a talkative mood, so I spoke up and explained we were there to see if she could prescribe some therapy to help in his recovery from the pelvic injury. She had his thick medical file with her, so I hoped she'd seen from his chart that he had a hairline fracture of the pelvis.

"Well, there's certainly no chance that I will prescribe any type of physical therapy without a complete physical, referral to an orthopedic specialist, and x-rays, plus anything else I feel is necessary to establish the best standard of care." *Was she actually glaring at me?* I thought as she delivered her curt response. Perhaps she had a point about establishing the best standard of care, but her delivery set me on edge.

I quickly learned that my attempt to dialogue with this physician was hopeless, as we were not going to see eye-to-eye when it came to my father's care. I wasn't willing to subject my dad to a multi-doctor odyssey, and it was obvious she wasn't going to budge in her declaration. If we wanted physical therapy for Dad, we would have to abide by her rigid rules and regulations. We ended the visit with me saying we'd get back to her later. I couldn't wait to leave, as the longer we were there, the more it felt like all the air was being sucked out of the room; if we stayed much longer, we might pass out. This was undoubtedly the worst experience I'd ever had with a physician.

Dad and I gratefully left the exam room and headed back to the waiting room to call for transport back to Tendercare Cottages. I sat there feeling defeated, with a sickening feeling that I'd made an impulsive and poorly informed decision to move my parents to this new medical facility. I again felt overwhelmed by the burden of parenting my parents. My dad didn't receive physical therapy, and I went through the process of transferring their medical records back to the original physician's office, where they would ultimately see one of their former internist's partners. This experience taught me the importance of patient/physician/family caregiver rapport, and to not assume either the physician's specialty or proximity to an eldercare facility automatically ensures they are the right choice.

Despite no physical therapy, Dad slowly began to recover. A seat belt with a lock was installed on his wheelchair. He started eating again. Most days found Dad sitting in his wheelchair with his chin resting on his chest and his eyes closed. He looked like he was sleeping, and sometimes he was, but not always. Often, he was actually listening, and sometimes his head slowly popped up and he'd say something lucid and right-on. Whenever it happened, it caught me off-guard and always amazed me. Typically, he didn't recognize me, usually positing that I was his "aunt" or "cousin." If I told him who I was, he seemed to know me, at least for that particular visit. My mother loved to ask him, "Who am I?" Often, he would say, "You are my aunt," or, "You are my mother." Sometimes this upset her, and sometimes she just laughed and said, "I knew I shouldn't have married you."

Because of the enjoyment he received from masturbation, it was common to find him with his hand down his pants. Or, if his prostate was bothering him, he spent time attempting to place his penis in a more comfortable position inside his briefs. Mom was very aware of where he liked to keep his hands, as several times she asked me what we could do about what she called his "thing."

"We need to do something about your dad's thing."

The first time she said this, I wondered incredulously to myself, *is she talking about what I think she is talking about?*

"Uh, what do you mean, Mom?" I replied.

"Well, it is too long. I think if we could cut if off a little shorter, it wouldn't bother him so much."

Oh my! Where does she get these ideas?

Trying to sound rational, as well as matter-of-fact, I said, "Mom, if we were to cut it off shorter, he wouldn't be able to urinate. He needs it all." In no uncertain terms, I added, "We cannot cut *any* of it off," hoping this would end the discussion.

I am not sure she was convinced, and then she threw in her zinger, "It must be so long because he is part Indian. I knew I should never have married him."

"What do you mean, 'part Indian?'" I asked her, perplexed. She was unable to explain, but reiterated it several times over a period of weeks. *What did she mean about him being "part Indian?" We'll never know.* In any case, to ward off a potential disaster, I found myself looking for, and removing, any scissors and table knives she might accidentally have in her room.

Speaking of scissors, Dad was not to be thwarted with the locked seatbelt on his wheelchair. One afternoon I received a call from Tendercare Cottages.

"Hi, I'm calling about your dad. He found a pair of scissors and cut his seat belt in half."

My dad knew what he wanted, and it was not to be confined to a wheelchair. Little did he know that he now had buy a new seatbelt! I hoped from now on that Tendercare Cottages kept a better watch on their scissors.

Dad loved wearing hats. It was unusual to see him without a hat of some sort, whether a straw hat, a baseball cap, or a fedora. One afternoon, as I sat and watched him roll around his room in his wheelchair, I wondered what he was thinking. He was hatless that afternoon, but not for long. Two baseball caps were sitting on his dresser; one was turquoise with a dolphin on it, and the other was red and in white lettering said, "Jim's Auto." I had no idea where either hat actually came from, as I hadn't given them to him. He wheeled over to pick up the turquoise hat, and after examining it, put it on. He looked at his reflection in the mirror, and I could tell by the look on his face that something wasn't quite right. Suddenly, his face lit up when he noticed the other red cap, which he promptly picked up and rested somewhat askew on top of the first cap. "Ah, this is just right," I imagined him thinking. He wheeled off through the doorway into the common area, forgetting entirely that I was sitting on his bed visiting with him.

My father's eating habits soon became an obsession for my mother. At Cedar Grove, it was evident whenever the three of us shared a meal together that she liked to nag him at mealtimes. This was nothing new, really, as I remember her criticizing his eating habits for many years in their home.

"Sit up. Lean forward. You make a mess, dropping bits of food in your lap. What is wrong with you?"

Her comments brought me back to our last meal together in Nelson City. I remembered his bib and the plastic mat under the kitchen table to catch his crumbs. Because coordination is often an issue for someone suffering from Parkinson's disease, it was more difficult for Dad to keep the food balanced on the fork or spoon, and some of it invariably ended up on his clothing or bib. Obsessed with cleanliness, Mom took these mishaps as a personal affront designed to cause her grief, not able to understand that he couldn't help it.

Because they were normally separated in different dining rooms at Cedar Grove, the move to Tendercare Cottages provided them the opportunity to eat meals together again, though in reality this never came to pass. The caregivers at Tendercare Cottages quickly discovered during my parents' very first meal, within an hour of their arrival at Tendercare Cottages, that my mother loved to badger my father, telling him to sit up, eat more, eat less, and wipe his mouth, fingers, or face. At the next and all subsequent meals, she was placed at a separate table, much like quarreling children separated in the lunchroom. Dad wasn't even "safe" at the other table. It was not uncommon for Mom to finish her meal and go over to his table to pester him. One day she even pulled him away from his meal, telling him he was "done." Trying to counter Mom's tiresome behavior, the caregivers began to serve his meal first before anyone else, as he ate very slowly. They served my mother last, in the hope that he would be close to finishing by the time that she was done eating. That was the plan, which kept her from wending her way over to his table to pester him while he ate. As long as Mom was actually occupied with her meal, this approach was successful.

Lesson Learned

Do not assume that because a physician is listed as specializing in geriatrics he or she will automatically be a good fit. Request an interview with the physician before committing your loved one to his/her care.

TWENTY-NINE
Scare

Mom had her first "incident" at the end of their third summer in Coulson. Jody, the night staff worker at Tendercare Cottages, called me around dinnertime. "Hello, Vicki? Your mother may have had a stroke. Her pulse is quite weak, and we wondered what you'd like us to do." In some sort of shock, I reacted without thinking, "Call an ambulance! We'll meet you at the hospital emergency department!"

Has mom really had a stroke? She has only a faint pulse? What does that mean? Is she dying? Wait, I am not ready for this. I didn't say goodbye! These were some of the thoughts that passed through my mind as I sat in the hospital emergency department waiting for the ambulance to arrive. Tears welled up in my eyes as I realized how life as we know it can change in a single instant.

While in the emergency room, Mom was subjected to more than four hours of tests. She repeatedly said, "I feel fine. Can we please go home now?" Lionel and I did our best to placate and comfort her, as my mind raced with thoughts of her imminent and sudden death. The preliminary tests found nothing conclusive, but the physician decided to keep her overnight in the hospital and do a few more tests. She stayed in the hospital for two days, and had more than $8,900 of tests including heart monitoring, an EEG, EKG/ECG, echocardiogram, two cat-scans, x-rays, and blood work. The physician indicated to me that the CT scan of Mom's brain showed signs of vascular dementia. I wasn't sure what this meant in relation to Alzheimer's disease, and because I was preoccupied with paranoid thoughts about my mother dying, I didn't immediately pursue further information about the vascular dementia.

On a positive note, Mom loved the hospital setting and all the attention. On one of my visits to her bedside, she asked me, "How much would it cost for your dad and me to move to this place? I really like it here!" She didn't understand that she was in the hospital.

Thanksgiving approached and since her hospital stay, Mom had had four additional "incidents." These incidents ranged from non-responsive fainting behavior to epileptic-type seizures. The first incident was the only one that included a hospital stay, as after that, a *Comfort One* measure was put into place for both my parents. This was a legal document provided by the local hospital and signed by me, as legal representative of both my parents, to indicate that they did not want any heroic measures taken on their behalf in the wake of a life-debilitating event. *Comfort One* stipulated that they receive palliative care only, which both illustrated and honored their choices spoken to me on many occasions in the past, and which they thought would be covered by their "living will." It wasn't.

I realized that calling the ambulance for Mom during that first incident was a gut reflex, a sort of panic-induced decision. Had I been more in control of all my mental faculties, I may not have made that decision. Why had I subjected my mother to two days of endless tests? What if they *had* found a heart problem? Were we going to send her into surgery for a pacemaker? I think not. Once I had time for further reflection, I also realized the best care for either of them was palliative care; my goal was to keep them comfortable and minimize any pain. In the past several years, Mom indicated to me many times that she was ready to "go," and her thoughts had not deviated from that wish. I felt I honored that choice with my decision to refrain from medical interventions, other than pain control, plus helping her and Dad remain as comfortable as possible. To prolong their seemingly dismal existence was not the goal. I remembered a conversation we had shortly after I moved them to Coulson. My dad looked at me and asked, "How long do I have to live?" I looked back at him and said, "I don't know Dad. That's up to God." He looked back at me quizzically, almost as if he was pondering his timeline with God.

Most people, myself included, have lives outside of the caregiver role. Many of us have children of our own to take care of, whether young or grown. Even though my children were grown and on their own, it didn't mean that I didn't experience the trickle-down effect of *their* stress as they were learning to cope with the complexities and uncertainties in life. I considered myself fortunate that we maintained close relationships, and they felt comfortable calling me to discuss those complexities and uncertainties. This piece did, however, add to the overall stress we often feel as caregivers, so it's important for the caregiver to have a support system and down time. Some days, I awakened from a poor night of sleep feeling bleary-eyed and inadequate for the tasks at hand. I am thankful that Lionel was so supportive through it all, and that I was often able to grab a quick nap sometime during the day.

Lessons Learned

Talk to your loved one as soon as possible about his or her wishes regarding heroic measures to be taken in the event of an emergency or accident. Put his or her requests in writing. I learned it needed to be more than a living will. Most hospitals have a document available to be completed regarding these issues. In our city, it is called "Comfort One," and states no heroic measures are to be taken. In keeping with Mom's wishes, we subsequently signed and put the Comfort One document into effect shortly after her first incident.

Remember to think before acting on impulse. Be sure that calling an ambulance and the subsequent hospitalization and tests are in alignment with your loved one's wishes.

Important note: you need downtime! It is easy to forget to take time for *yourself!* Taking time to rest and rejuvenate is extremely important!

THIRTY
Daily Living

I arrived at my mother's apartment at 2 p.m. one afternoon. Upon knocking and hearing her invitation to come in, I opened the door and was greeted with her shocked face, as if she couldn't fathom why I was there. She cautiously ventured, "What are you doing here? It's time for bed." As my focus returned, I realized my mother was sitting in front of me, on her bed, completely naked.

"Look outside," I replied as gently as I could, "Is it dark out?"

She turned and gazed out her window at the clear, azure blue sky. "No," she replied, matter-of-factly.

"You can go to bed when it gets dark outside, okay?"

I was immediately struck with the same recurring thought that, in so many ways, dealing with demented people is like living with toddlers.

On another visit, Mom was having trouble locating the tissues that she had placed in her pants pockets. Upon further observation, I realized it was because she had her elastic-waist jeans on backwards and couldn't reach the pockets!

The administrator at Tendercare Cottages informed me that following a move to a new facility, it takes the elderly about 90 days to adjust. It had been more than 90 days, and Mom had still not adjusted. If anything, the move to Tendercare Cottages seemed to have *accelerated* Mom's decline, as her dementia was more and more noticeable. The latest development was her declaration she could no longer read.

"There is no sense in bringing me any more magazines. I can't read anymore," she said with resignation in her voice.

What could I possibly say in response to that? I looked at her with compassion, but couldn't stop thinking about how one of her few remaining pleasures was now fleeting. I supposed I no longer needed to continue the search for her eyeglasses, which had mysteriously gone missing.

On many days, the activities coordinator at Tendercare Cottages drew Mom into crafts and bingo, and my parents still enjoyed the weekly bus rides and sporadic musical entertainment; most days, however, were an endless number of minutes, breaths, and gazes spent waiting for the next meal, or to go to bed. My mother continued her nighttime "exhibitionist" behavior, usually showing up in the common room naked, and cursing like a drunken sailor stumbling out of a seaside tavern. The inhibitions that once formed the fabric of my mother's politesse were clearly diminishing. Shoving the caregivers, hiding her laundry, and refusing to shower or change her underwear became her new norm. Each day and night brought fresh challenges.

One day when visiting her, I decided we'd look at one of their photo albums for something to do to pass the time. My expectations were dashed when each picture became a repetitious reminder of my mother's memory loss. We looked at a picture together and I identified the people. Then we moved on to the next picture, quite similar to the previous photo, and I again identified the people. Now, to some extent I don't mind repeating myself, but by the tenth page, when my eyes had glazed over, I began to feel crazy. *Is this what dementia is like?* My mother is still identifying herself as me, or me as herself. She couldn't remember from one picture to the next who it was, so we cycled through an endless iteration of, "Is this me?" with a pause, then, "Is this you?" I realized this activity was stressful for both of us, and made a mental note to myself not to repeat it. Despite this, I was heartened that she could remember who her grandkids were when their pictures were identified each time.

Lessons Learned

It can be very agitating to someone with Alzheimer's to participate in activities that make his or her memory loss apparent, not to mention the frustration it can cause you, the caregiver. My innocent idea to peruse Mom's photo albums backfired, as I realized she could no longer identify her friends, relatives, or even herself in photos. Try not to ask someone with moderately severe Alzheimer's open-ended questions, such as, "Who am I?" or "Who is that?"

Anne Basting, Ph.D., founder of the creative storytelling program TimeSlips (www.timeslips.org) has utilized storytelling as a therapeutic activity for individuals with dementia. Your loved one is shown a picture and asked to tell an improvised story about what's happening in it. It is a low-stress way to encourage them to communicate and doesn't rely on memory. A study published in *Nursing Research* found people who participated in this program were happier and better able to communicate.

THIRTY-ONE
Odd Conversations

After the move to the new facility, I changed the pattern of calling Mom each day, more for my own sanity than anything else. In the beginning, I called her room several times a week, but by late fall, the conversations had taken a turn for the bizarre, and I realized the calls were not positive for either of us. She told me the most peculiar things.

"Hi, Mom."

"Oh, I wanted to tell you that a man called," Mom announced one evening.

"A man called you? What man?" I questioned her.

"You know, the man who has taken care of me for the past year."

"Gosh, Mom, I don't know who you mean. What did he say?" My mind was racing to figure out who or what she was talking about.

"Well, he told me things would be better."

"That's good." I wondered if this was something important and she didn't understand what he meant or needed. *Maybe it was a wrong number? Who was "he?" Then, the unsettling thought, did "he" even exist?*

"Yes, and he also told me, by the way, that I could eat the peaches."

I suppose my last questions may have been answered, but I'll never know for sure.

Despite her declining communicative skills, Mom could still repeat a long litany of complaints about Tendercare Cottages, which didn't do either of us any good. It became more difficult for me to call her. Word retrieval was a constant issue, and she had difficulty forming sentences, so she was usually unable to say what she wanted. There were still some rare occasions when her speech magically reappeared, however temporary or fantastical it might have been. I spent the majority of our conversations guessing about what she meant, and she spent them feeling frustrated, unable to communicate her wishes. It was much like talking with a toddler who knows what he or she wants to say, but doesn't yet have the vocabulary to say it. The outcome was often a temper tantrum. The simple solution for me was to stop calling Mom as frequently. While I thought this might make it easier on me, Mom actually seemed to be cognizant of my infrequent calls, and often cried to me, "You never call me any more." I found myself caught between a rock and a hard place.

One call began with a fall from her chair as she attempted to answer the phone. Instead of hearing "hello," I heard a muffled cry and a thudding sound. Several long seconds later, I finally heard a faint "Hello?"

"Hi Mom. Are you okay?"

"I think so. The darn chair just fell over with me in it! Say, I forgot to have you do the itch when you were here last."

"Oh. Do you mean I forgot to scratch your back?"

"Maybe."

"Well, I can ask the caregiver to scratch your back for you."

"Oh no, it's fine."

Silence.

"Uh, have you seen Dad today?"

"Oh, yes."

"How is he today?"

"Oh fine. I laid down with him today."

"Oh, you did? On his bed?"

"No. On the flat thing. You know what I mean."

I was puzzled. "Do you mean in the recliner?"

"Yeah, I think so."

"Did you both lay in the same one? Was it a little crowded?" I chuckled.

"No. Oh, I don't know where it was."

By now I'm thinking maybe she dreamt it. *Let's see,* I am thinking to myself as the silence draws on, *I can't talk about the food because she'll start complaining, and I can't talk about what I've been doing because she gets jealous, hmm … maybe the weather …*

"So, it's about 45 degrees out. We are going to go take a walk, even though it isn't very warm." *Shoot! I forgot and said something about myself.*

In a sarcastic voice, she retorted, "Well, that must be nice," seeming to imply "here I am, stuck in this facility."

"Will you tell Dad hello for me?"

Relief evident in her voice, "Yes, I'll do that right now."

Relieved, I answered, "Great. Well, talk to you later."

"Okay, goodbye."

"Bye."

Was it better to call and struggle, or was it better to not call and deal with hurt feelings when she says I never call? There appeared to be no easy answer to this dilemma.

My visits were at least once a week, and during them I had the opportunity to practice the art of being. With Mom's word retrieval issues and Dad's perpetual dozing, it was difficult to carry on a conversation with either one of them. We did, however, repeat any topic that she *did* want to talk about. She developed an obsession with her clock.

"Is my clock set correctly?"

"Yes Mom, I set it the last time I was here."

Not yet a minute later, "Is my clock set correctly?"

"Yes Mom, I set it the last time I was here."

Within another minute, she would again ask "Is my clock set correctly?"

"Yes Mom, I set it the last time I was here."

"Is my clock set correctly?"

Changing tactics: "Yes Mom, I set it the last time I was here, but why don't we check it again together?"

And so it went.

I became very proficient at repeating statements with a gentle, kind voice, which was not always my *forte* at the beginning of our dementia journey. I sometimes remembered my exasperation over the whole issue of her operating, or not operating, her computer. It seemed like a lifetime ago to me, not just a few years.

The new ritual was tweezing errant hairs from her face.

"Hi Mom, how are you today?"

"Did you bring the tweezers?"

"Yes, here they are," I said as I pulled the tweezers out of my pocket. Because she often misplaced or sometimes threw away little items from her drawers, I kept her tweezers in my car and brought them in with me when I visited her. Our usual routine consisted of her lying on the bed with her head positioned close to the window above. This position shed more light on the stiff, exasperating little hairs that she rubbed her fingers over saying, "Pull here, pull here."

In an odd sort of way, I found this little ritual a concrete way to be able to do something that pleased her, as well as a way to offer my love through human touch.

Lessons Learned

I cannot reiterate enough the importance of exercising patience and kindness when dealing with your loved one. Don't be impatient when asked to repeat things, and try to respond gently when the same question is repeated over and over again. If you are able, try to gently change the subject.

In connection with this lesson, I have also learned what is called the 10-second rule, which applies to communicating with someone suffering from Alzheimer's. This means that because people with Alzheimer's disease do not process things as well, or as quickly as people not suffering from dementia, we should give a 10-second pause after we ask a question for them to respond. If they don't respond, we can then repeat it, but it should be repeated using the same phrasing, so as not to confuse them further.

When I remembered to use it, this rule was helpful. There were times, however, that my question was met with a vacant stare and it seemed to drift gently unanswered into space.

Do not discount the power of touch as a way to bond with your loved one when all other methods seem futile. I learned to be creative with the power of touch by tweezing Mom's errant facial hairs with a gentle hand. Understand that sometimes, just sitting quietly together is time well-spent. Remember that there may not be much opportunity for loving touch, so plan on holding hands whenever you visit.

THIRTY-TWO
Food Issues

Food continued to be a problem for my mother. That autumn, she called me several times in three days to tell me that the caregivers at Tendercare Cottages were ruining her meals so she couldn't eat them.

"We have to do something about the food in this place!" Mom exclaimed again. "They slop water on my food and ruin it. I can't begin to eat it. You should see it! It makes me gag. They just don't know how to cook!"

I thought perhaps it was gravy or a soupy casserole that was bothering her. By the end of the second day of repeated calls, though, I began to be suspicious. As always when it came to Mom, I had difficulty sorting whether what she told me was fantasy, truth, or something in between. It turns out it was something in between.

On the third day, I called and visited with the caregivers.

"Hi. Mom seems to be having some trouble with the food. Have you been having a lot of casseroles lately?"

"No, but your mother is having some problems at mealtimes," offered the caregiver. "She often puts her food in her water glass or pours her drinks onto her food, or just dumps her drink on the table. Yesterday she scooped up some food and smeared it all across the table and under her fingernails. She appeared to be thoroughly enjoying herself, and was obviously not interested in eating."

Another day, when I talked to Mom, she reported, "They won't let me have tea to drink any more. They don't know how to make it anyways. It's always cold."

When I followed up on that, I was told, "Your Mom leaves the tea until it has turned cold, and then gets angry and upset that it isn't hot, and often dumps it over. We don't want her to injure herself if she tips it over and it *is* hot, so we haven't given her any tea these last few days. She doesn't ever seem to drink it anyway."

Against all logic, part of me wanted to believe, at least in some way, the things she told me. I again realized that I must question everything she reported and recognize that her stories were probably exaggerated and turned around, usually involving blaming her own behavior on the caregivers, or that stories she told me were simply imagined.

I placed a call to her psychiatrist, Dr. Nielson, who, upon hearing what was happening, determined that Mom had a component of Alzheimer's called Sundowner's Effect. This essentially meant she turned into a very different person when evening arrived, hence the derivation of the name. Sundowner's Effect is thought to be a sleep or mood disorder, which can cause extreme agitation, irritability, and/or confusion, usually during the late afternoon or early evening hours. Stress or drug interactions associated with lower cognitive function may be responsible for this behavior, although this theory is not medically conclusive. Sundowner's Effect is often a characteristic of someone suffering from moderate to severe dementia. The psychiatrist adjusted her medication, which improved life for everyone.

Mom's issues with food accelerated, and she began to obsessively fixate on the food's shortcomings.

"The toast here is mushy."

"The toast here is too dark and hard to eat."

"The toast here is too dry and sticks to my mouth, and I can't swallow it."

My mother loved toast, so complaints often centered on this particular food item. The other 15 residents, including my dad, ate without any difficulty. When I visited, I often heard Mom ask Dad, "What do you think of the food?" His reply was, "Very good." Her comeback, "Well, I'm always wrong. I might as well go jump in the river." For whatever reason, drowning was her suicidal preference. My mother suffered from poor self-esteem, and with the disease, her self-deprecating tendencies were only magnified. She began refusing to eat, or ate only very little, complaining loudly about the "awful" food the caregivers served.

Mealtimes evolved into a series of endless complaints, including, "The man next to me smells and I can't eat," so they moved her to a different seat at the table.

"Having to sit with this table full of people is killing me, and I can't eat sitting next to them," so they fed her before or after everyone else so she could be alone—and there could not be *anyone* left at the table before she came out of her room to eat.

"Looking at food makes me feel sick."

"The food here is sloppy, mushy, and sickening."

"You just have *no* idea how bad the food is."

"These young girls do not know how to cook."

The list went on and on. When I joined her for a meal, the food tasted fine to me; she looked at me with incredulity, hardly able to believe I had eaten the food. She said, "Well, maybe it is me. There is something wrong with me."

I think she was right. There was something wrong with her. Perhaps her taste buds had changed, and the food no longer tasted good to her, or maybe it was her body's way of shutting down at the end stages of life. Should we have done a series of diagnostic tests? She simply didn't want to eat. She complained of having no energy, and wanted to lie on her bed a lot of the time. Should we have allowed her to do that, or should we have cajoled her into participating in eating, activities, and life? What was the right moral choice?

Lesson Learned

Remember to honor the wishes of your loved one. This may involve asking some difficult questions, particularly involving eating issues.

THIRTY-THREE
Hospice

One day when I arrived for a visit, I found Mom sitting on her bed. She looked at me tearfully, "Vicki, I just want to drop," she cried, depressed and despondent.

"Oh, Mom, I'm sorry. Are you frightened?"

She said emphatically with more strength in her voice, "No. I just feel lousy." I wasn't sure how to pursue this conversation further, let alone how to make her feel better. Where did my influence, my input, end? Should I have called her psychiatrist about what I had perceived as an abnormally low mood? Perhaps I had misinterpreted her comment, thinking she was talking about wanting to die when I had asked her if she was frightened. What would have been the best way to maneuver these situations? Was there something else I might have said? Once again, it was important to remember that Mom basically lived on a different plane of existence.

In light of this situation, a friend of mine shared with me her insights regarding Hospice, an organization that helps families cope with end-of-life issues. She felt I might want to call their office to see if my parents might be considered for their program. Three weeks later, my parents and I sat with Sally, a Hospice social worker, at a dining table at Tendercare Cottages. Sally asked many questions, and in an effort to discern my parents' cognitive abilities, she first directed the questions to them. The interview lasted about an hour. A few days later Hospice called to inform me that they'd completed their assessment.

"Unfortunately, at the present time your parents don't meet the necessary criteria to be admitted to Hospice. However, their applications will be kept on file in case their respective conditions worsen, in which case they would be reevaluated. As the social worker you visited with might have mentioned, to be accepted into Hospice means there is a strong possibility the applicant will pass away within six months, and your parents don't fit that criteria yet."

On the one hand this gave me a certain solace, but on the other hand …

How quickly a situation can change. Less than a month after the initial Hospice interview, Mom qualified for Hospice care after she lost 12 pounds in a period of just two weeks. She basically stopped eating. If she was somehow coerced into eating, she consumed very little. This initial weight loss was described as "failure to thrive," and was what prompted Tendercare Cottages' call to Hospice. It came as a surprise that the facility had arranged for Hospice care, notifying me only after the fact. On the other hand, it was also a relief to know Hospice was now on board to help with decisions and care. I learned from Linda, the Hospice nurse assigned to Mom's care, that yes, losing the desire to eat was a sign of the end stage of life. She told me that the body's metabolic rate decreases, and the thought of food seems to make the dying person nauseous. Was my mother's body just winding down, doing what comes naturally at the end of life, or was it something else? It's obviously not the food, or the cooking, as my mother wanted us to believe.

The situation changed again the following week, however, as Mom suddenly started eating again, and while she was not eating much, it was something. Some days she ate more than others, though at best, it was still notably minuscule portions: a tablespoon of food here, a teaspoon there, juice, water, and occasionally tea (they were carefully giving her tea again). Hospice said she could subsist on this diet for quite a long time. Our bodies are truly amazing, surviving on so little.

Lessons Learned

Find out what services are available from your local Hospice organization, and utilize them. Even though my parents didn't qualify for Hospice initially, learning about their services and knowing what was available if the situation deteriorated gave me a certain peace of mind. When the facility later contacted Hospice concerning Mom's deteriorating health, I was already familiar and comfortable with the organization and the types of assistance and care they offer.

PART TWO

My Fair Lady...

THIRTY-FOUR
Giving Thanks

Two weeks after Mom was admitted into Hospice, Thanksgiving Day arrived. When Lionel and I dropped by Tendercare Cottages for a visit, it was immediately apparent that Mom was in a foul mood. The caregiver informed us that Mom had fallen out of bed earlier and bumped her head on her night table. Fortunately, she seemed all right, other than a bruise on her temple.

For the last two weeks, Mom had been awakening most mornings in a pool of diarrhea. Because she insisted on removing the disposable underwear the facility had her wear at night, it made an already unpleasant cleanup that much worse. The caregivers looking after Mom had my undying appreciation. Today Pat, one of the caregivers, told me that after Mom's carpet was scrubbed and she was presentable, Mom spent the morning alone in her room, not wanting to eat breakfast or speak to anyone. Based on the chilly reception I received when we arrived, it was obvious Mom didn't want to speak to me today, either.

Avoiding eye contact, she said haughtily, "Well, nice you could make it. It's been, what, 50 days since you visited me?"

(*Sighing*) "Mom, I was here a week ago. That's seven days, not 50."

She glared at me with suspicion, obviously thinking I had made this up.

"Where have you been?" she asked pointedly, implying that we had been traveling *yet again* (a troubling subject for her).

At least she was actively addressing me now, which was better than when we first arrived, and she wouldn't even look at me.

"We have been at work and at home mostly," was my truthful reply, which earned me more glaring. I decided the best tactic at this point was to change the subject, and offered to call her grandchildren or my brother.

We called my son Kyle and daughter Megan, who were spending Thanksgiving together in Michigan, where Megan lives. Kyle goes to graduate school in Ohio, so I was glad they could get together for the holiday.

Conversations on the telephone had become difficult because of Mom's ever-declining word-retrieval ability, and the awkwardness of a one-sided conversation made today's call brief. After only a minute or two on the phone with Megan, there was a pause and I heard my daughter say, "Um, well, good to talk to you Grandma. You can talk to Kyle now."

With no sign of recognition, my mother said to Megan, "Who is Kyle?" After he came on the phone, she listened to him for a few minutes before asking, "So, how is your sister Megan?" This is what short-term memory loss was like.

Next, we called my brother Jack. This was another very short-lived conversation. After a minute or two, I could hear him asking to talk to me. When I put the phone to my ear, he asked me, "Did she tell you I called her two hours ago?"

"Uh, no," I replied. No wonder she thought it had been 50 days since I had last visited! My sense was that I could visit 50 times in 50 days, and she would still think I hadn't been to see her for a long time. I was reminded of the Drew Barrymore movie, *50 First Dates*, in which Barrymore's character wakes up each morning unaware of the fact that her memory has been erased. Maybe that's what life was like for Mom.

Mom's implicit accusation that I did not visit her often enough definitely pushed my buttons, and was an effective method of drowning me in guilt, even though I knew it wasn't true. The difficulty for me was realizing that no matter how much I attempted to "be there" for her, it was never going to be enough. Here was yet another reminder of how a rational brain can function irrationally when dealing with a demented loved one.

Lesson Learned

The concept of passing time can change drastically for someone with dementia, so remember this, and practice patience when dealing with him/her.

THIRTY-FIVE
"I Will Be Dead by Then"

It became customary during our phone conversations for Mom to express her irritation about the facility's food.

"Vicki, there's something wrong with my stomach, and I think it's from the food they give us. You just have *no* idea how awful it is."

"Mom, you have a doctor's appointment in five days, so we can visit with the doctor about your stomach then, okay?"

"Well, I will be dead by then," she snapped. Always a flair for the dramatic, that woman!

In addition to my parents' regular check-up, the primary mission at the forthcoming doctor's appointment was my request to administer the Mini Mental State Examination (MMSE) in order to check where Mom currently measured on the scale of Alzheimer's diagnoses. Given the dramatic changes in her behavior and abilities lately, my intuition was that her score would be close to zero. Because of this, I also planned to inquire about the merits of continuing her Alzheimer medications.

There is a helpful resource called the Alzheimer's Association Help Line, which has 24-hour telephone care (1-800-272-3900). I spoke with one of their social workers in advance of my parents' doctor's appointment, and she helped me sort through the pros and cons of either continuing or discontinuing Mom's Alzheimer's medications. I learned that if the MMSE determined that Mom had deteriorated—to severe dementia—it was likely the drugs were no longer serving a useful purpose. If this were the case, it was not worth continuing the medication due to the potential negative side effects, such as diarrhea, dizziness and falls, confusion, and agitation. It seemed to me she had all of these side effects, and if she now had severe dementia, discontinuing the medications might be the appropriate choice. The social worker explained that my questions and anxieties were common in this situation, which I found reassuring. She said my feelings were not unusual, as most caregivers struggle with the decision about when and if to stop the medications. Feelings of guilt and hopelessness were common reactions. It helped to know that I was not alone, and there were others out there who, like me, faced these sorts of questions and/or dilemmas on a daily basis. After discussing the situation with the social worker, I sensed the answer to my question concerning the Alzheimer's medications would be more apparent following the doctor's evaluation.

THIRTY-SIX
The Doctor Visit

MET Special Transit, a different company than my parents had used at Cedar Grove, was bringing them to their doctor's visit. I was instructed by Tendercare Cottages to meet my parents in the doctor's office lobby. This was their first appointment back at their previous doctor's office since they'd moved into their new assisted-living facility. I always felt anxious when I met my parents at their various appointments, fearful that I'd be late and they'd get lost. As such, I tended to arrive much too early, giving my anxiety more time to grow while I waited.

Today, as I apprehensively awaited their arrival in the lobby of the third floor doctor's office, I looked at the clock and discovered it was five minutes past the agreed-upon arrival time, and they weren't there. It seemed unlike Tendercare Cottages to be late. After 10 minutes had passed, I called the facility, only to learn the special transport had left there with my parents 15 minutes prior. Where were they? I felt panic begin to wash over me. Suddenly (and not a moment too soon), the main floor lobby receptionist appeared asking if anyone knew what had happened to the family member (me) who was supposed to meet the elderly couple in the main entrance lobby. I had incorrectly assumed that because Tendercare Cottages had instructed me to meet them in the *doctor's office* lobby, that they would actually bring them there and not just drop them off in the *main* lobby. Feeling frazzled, I quickly retrieved my parents from the main lobby, and we took the elevator back to the third floor doctor's office. Although seemingly insignificant, this incident intensified my accumulated stress and anxiety as caregiver.

After waiting for several minutes, the nurse called us back to the exam room. As we maneuvered down the hallway with Mom's walker and Dad's wheelchair, I knew the first stop would be at the scales in order to do a weight check. My father was difficult to lift out of his wheelchair, so we usually skipped his weight, and today was no exception. The doctor normally eyeballed him and determined whether his weight was within a normal range, which it easily was. Mom, on the other hand, had lost six pounds since her last visit with the doctor five months ago, and was down 12 pounds from the visit before that. Of course, before she stepped on the scale, she announced, "Well, I've lost about 50 pounds because of the bad food." I rolled my eyes. After the weigh-in, we meandered further down the hall; from prior experience, I recognized it was best to first back Dad's chair into the postage stamp-sized room, then squeeze Mom and myself into the two padded, wooden exam room chairs. The exam table easily took up a third of the room, which did not leave a lot of additional space. Even though a tight fit, we had quickly learned it's easier for everyone to be in one room than for me to attempt to keep tabs on each of them in two different rooms. The nurse somehow managed to cram herself into the room with us. Thankfully, no one was claustrophobic. She measured their blood pressure while Mom started rambling, "The food's just awful. I don't know how they could expect anyone to eat it." I think I looked at the nurse and rolled my eyes again, imploring her to understand. Both had excellent blood pressure readings, with Mom's blood pressure 97 over 60 and Dad's 108 over 70.

Thankfully, the doctor quickly arrived, greeted us, and began his exam. He started with Mom, and went through a review of all her medications. Next, he began the MMSE evaluation.

"I'm going to ask you some questions now if that's okay."

"Uh huh."

"Can you tell me what year it is?"

"No."

"Can you tell me what month it is?"

"No."

"Can you tell me what day it is?"

"No."

"Can you tell me what season it is?"

"Hmm," (struggling to pull up the word) "hmm…half-day?"

"Can you tell me what kind of building we're in?"

"No."

"Okay, then, I'm going to say three words to you and I would like you to repeat them. We'll then wait 30 to 45 seconds, and I'll ask you to repeat them to me again, okay?"

"Okay."

"Red, car, love."

"Red, car, love," repeated Mom.

"Yes, red, car, love."

"Red, car, love," repeated Mom for a second time.

"Very good! We'll come back to that. Can you spell 'world' for me?"

"W-O-R-L-D."

"That's right! Now, can you spell 'world' backwards for me?"

"Oh, no."

"Okay, then … now, what were the three words?"

"I don't know."

The doctor wrote "close your eyes" on a piece of paper and showed it to her. "Can you do this?"

Mom read it aloud, "Close your eyes."

"Yes, can you do what it says?"

Mom read it aloud again, "Close your eyes."

"Yes, can you do that?"

Mom squeezed her eyes shut.

"Very good! Now, what is this I'm holding?" (He held up a pen.)

"A pencil."

He clicked the pen several times. "What is this?"

"A pencil."

"Could you write a sentence for me?"

"Oh no, I can't write."

"Okay, then. Let's see."

He looked at me and said, "Well, it looks like she scored a four."

She scored a four out of a possible 30 points. That confirmed an anticipated score of near zero, but it didn't make it any less heartbreaking to witness this very obvious, dramatic decline.

The first time my mother had this test administered was in Nelson City when she was originally diagnosed with Alzheimer's a little over three years ago; at that time, she was able to write and even draw a little; she scored an 18. The test was repeated after they moved to Coulson, and I was there to watch. She struggled, but was still able to successfully write, and she scored a 15. The following year, a year before this day, her score was a 12. Going from a score of 12 to four was by far the most significant decline to date, and was evidence of the advanced progression of her disease. What was once moderate Alzheimer's was now classified as severe. Not surprisingly, her doctor recommended discontinuing her two Alzheimer's medications, Aricept and Namenda. I agreed with him, as it was apparent the medications were no longer helping Mom's memory and were potentially causing side effects.

Seemingly out of nowhere, my mother exclaimed to the doctor, "You know, I feel like I need to push. I keep feeling like I want to have a bowel movement."

"Do you feel that way right now?" he asked.

"Of course! I feel this way all the time now."

"Hmm," he looked at me and said, "I think I'll take her into the exam room next door, if that's okay, because she may have an impaction."

I quickly gave permission, and the doctor helped my mother to the door. As they were leaving, Dad looked at me, smiled, and said shyly, "What is that woman's name?" It was obvious he was "interested" in her, and wanted to find out who she was.

"That's Trudy. She's your wife."

He smiled happily, obviously not fully comprehending what "wife" meant, and asked, "What's her last name?" I could tell he was definitely going to follow up on this!

After a few minutes of companionable silence, he looked at me and shared, "With all this talk about BMs, I'd like to have a bowel movement myself." I asked him if he could please wait a bit, and hoped the doctor and Mom would hurry back. They returned and I saw Dad's face light up when she walked through the door, the BM apparently forgotten. The doctor said, "Hey, Romeo, we're back. That's what your wife is calling you," he added. Dad smiled broadly.

Mom had no impaction, but the doctor requested some blood work on her before we left. She complained some more about her stomach and the food. She said, "Ever since those four girls came, it's been bad. They have no business cooking when they don't know anything about it." The "girls" were the same caregivers that cooked when she thought the food was fabulous in those first couple of months after moving there. She looked at me and implored, "Can't you move us somewhere where they know how to cook?"

The doctor suggested we add an antacid to her list of medications in the hope that it would settle her stomach. He thought her upset stomach might be a reaction to the pain medication she took for her arthritis. This might make sense, since he discontinued the antacid when she was in the hospital a couple of months ago, and she had stopped eating shortly thereafter.

We also discovered, from her medication list, that she was being given a daily stool softener. This was news to me, or perhaps with all the stress, I had simply forgotten. "I think we can safely remove the stool softener from her medication list," the doctor noted. It was no wonder she was having daily diarrhea! I was surprised that the nurse at the facility, or the Hospice nurse, hadn't noticed this. Her medication list was now reduced to four pills: an antidepressant, the drug to counteract paranoia and the Sundowner's Effect, a pain medication for arthritis, and the newly added antacid.

Next was Dad's turn for a general checkup. Lungs good, heart good, no pain to speak of. The doctor ordered blood work to check Dad's fluctuating sodium level.

Finally, we went down the hall to the lab to have blood drawn for both of them. This went smoothly, and then we were finished. We took the elevator down to the reception desk, where the receptionist called for special transport to retrieve them. We were informed the wait time for pickup could be anywhere from 10 minutes to an hour. To pass the time, I helped the receptionist hang some streamers on the Christmas tree she was decorating in the lobby next to where my parents were waiting. *Would this be my mother's last Christmas?* My mind couldn't shake this thought as we carefully draped the shimmering silver streamers across the tree. Apparently the approaching holiday did not register with either Mom or Dad as they sat waiting for the bus; if it did, they gave no acknowledgement.

Luckily, today we only waited around 20 minutes for the special transport bus. Once my parents were safely loaded onto the bus, I took a refreshing, brisk walk home.

A week later, both of their blood work came back completely fine, although Dad continued to suffer from mild anemia.

THIRTY-SEVEN
The Mysterious "White Thing"

It was an early December evening and I was relaxing in my living room, curled up by fireplace with a good book in hand when the phone rang.

"Hello?"

"Hi. You wouldn't believe it!"

"Hi, Mom. Wouldn't believe what?"

"When I got back from supper, I went to go to the bathroom, and found this white thing stuck to my gut!"

"Really? What do you mean? Can you tell me more about it?"

"Well, I think maybe we need to call the doctor. I've never seen anything like it before."

"Do you think that it's food that got inside your pants or something, and stuck to you? Maybe it's a sugar cookie, or a piece of potato?" (I struggled to think of what she could have eaten that was white.)

"No, it isn't. It's warm and I saved it."

Uh oh, I suddenly had a bad feeling about this.

"Hmm, was it inside your underpants?"

"No, it was stuck to my gut."

"Mom, let me call the caregiver and have her come help you."

We hung up and I called the Tendercare Cottages phone number. By now, I was fairly certain what it was, but it shouldn't be white! *Has Mom now also lost the ability to iden-*

tify colors? When Jody answered the phone, I explained what Mom was telling me, and asked if she could check on her. Jody said she'd call me back. Several minutes went by and my telephone rang again.

"Oh, my goodness, it was a piece of her bowel movement!" exclaimed Jody.

"Was it really white?"

"No, it was the normal color. I flushed it down the toilet, and explained to her what it was, but I'm not sure she grasped the idea."

Jody washed my mother's hands, and Mom called me back. I could hear her voice in the distance, but it was obvious she couldn't hear me very well. I realized that was because she must have been holding the phone upside down. In a loud voice, I shouted, "Mom, turn the phone around!" and once she did that and could hear me, I was able to reassure her that what she had found in her pants was a normal part of a bowel movement. Maybe since she had had so much diarrhea lately, she was no longer familiar with what a normal bowel movement resembled. She insisted she had never seen anything like it before, and couldn't understand where it had come from.

We had now moved into even scarier territory.

THIRTY-EIGHT
Medical Mishaps

"Hello, Vicki? This is Shelly, the nurse from Tendercare. I wanted to let you know that your mom has fallen six times in the past 72 hours, including falling out of bed twice."

"Oh, no! That's awful! Is she okay?"

"Well, there aren't any signs of broken bones, but she's definitely got some bruising on her face, arms, and legs. We've decided to move her mattress onto the floor in order to shorten the distance she falls."

"That seems like a wise idea," I wholeheartedly agreed.

"She's also experiencing a lot of night energy! We're having trouble keeping her in bed. We usually find her walking around naked at least once a night," Shelly sighed, and went on to say, "She smeared feces all over the floor of her room again last night, which means another carpet shampooing."

I interrupted her, "Oh, my gosh! I'm so sorry!"

"Oh, no, don't feel bad. That's just part of the job here. We're also concerned that she's had two more incidents that I can't describe other than falling asleep while standing up, and then kind of collapsing onto the ground. The reason I'm bringing all this up is because we're wondering if it all might be related to stopping the meds she takes for paranoia and Sundowner's Effect for that week, and then re-starting them."

Whaaat?

"Excuse me, what did you say?"

"Yes, we ran out of the meds the week before last, so when we called her primary care doctor, he told us to just stop giving them to her until he saw her for her appointment on the 28th. We got orders to restart them that day after she had her appointment."

"I'm sorry. I'm very confused by this. Why didn't anyone call me? What do you mean she was out of those meds?" I was doing my best to keep my voice under control, all the while feeling a rising sense of incredulous frustration. "I order her medications through the mail, and I know for a fact you couldn't have run out, because I always order a three-month supply. There should have been at least one month's worth left! There must have been some sort of mistake," my voice trailed off.

"Really? I don't know what happened then. All I can tell you is that the pharmacy told us they were out of the med, so I guess whoever was staffing that day forgot you ordered her meds. Then, when we called the doctor, he wouldn't refill the prescription until he saw her. After her appointment with him, he told us to go ahead and re-start the medication. Since we've been having so many problems with her this last week, and think it might be related, we've put in a call to her doctor for permission to stop them again."

I was completely caught off-guard. Evidently, the cascading series of events began when the pharmacy mistakenly thought they were out of the medication. Tendercare Cottages was simply following protocol when they called Mom's primary care physician, who didn't know that I ordered her medications through mail order. Although I was upset, I made every effort to keep my cool and not start pointing fingers, as I knew that wouldn't accomplish anything. This situation had suddenly become a very serious incident, with the full extent of the unfortunate repercussions for Mom not yet apparent.

"Shelly, before you stop the medication again, I'd like to speak to Dr. Nielson, her psychiatrist, who was the original ordering physician. Please don't do anything until I speak with her." I made this appeal before ending the conversation.

It was my feeling that Dr. Nielson should be involved in this decision-making process. I was extremely concerned about what might happen if my mother discontinued this medication again. All I could do was call and leave a message for Dr. Nielson, and hope she would call me back soon.

The phone was ringing when I walked in the back door after running my errands. I rushed to the phone.

"Hello?"

"Hello, Vicki. This is Linda from Hospice. I wanted to check in with you after my visit with your mom yesterday afternoon." I usually didn't know about these visits until after the fact. She went on to say "Your mom has lost another pound in the past week, and the caregivers are still having problems with her smearing food around the plate and across the table. If she does eat, it is very, very little."

She continued, "Three nights ago, after much encouragement to try the cream of broccoli soup, she actually swallowed two spoonfuls, but not surprisingly, left her muffin and fruit cocktail untouched. The caregiver I spoke with said they all chuckled when, after those two sips of soup, your mom looked up and said it was the 'best damn meal' she'd ever eaten. She's quite unpredictable!"

"Oh gosh. She continues to be a handful, doesn't she?"

"Well, in some ways. It's all part of the disease."

"Linda, I'm glad you called," I changed the subject, and explained what had happened with the medication mix-up.

"Oh, that's so unfortunate! I had no idea. Hmm … well, that *might* explain her current behavior, but I am inclined to think it has more to do with her deteriorating condition, and not solely the medication snafu."

"I hope you're right, and we haven't made her worse with this mix-up," I fretted. "I feel so frustrated that the chain of communication has these gaps, and that Mom's having to go through this." Sharing my concerns with Linda helped relieve my stress.

When Lionel came home for lunch, I explained to him what had happened with Mom's meds. Being a physician, he surmised something different altogether. He thought there was a possibility she might be suffering a series of small strokes. One thing was obvious: no one knew for sure what was going on.

As the day wore on, I anxiously awaited a return phone call from Dr. Nielson. Lionel and I were planning to attend the Christmas party for the residents and families of Tendercare Cottages that evening, so we would see Mom's current behavior/condition for ourselves.

Later in the afternoon, I called the facility to check on Mom. I was told she was making peculiar statements, and appeared quite drowsy from her night wanderings and lack of sleep. I still hadn't heard from Mom's psychiatrist by the time we left our house to drive to Tendercare Cottages. When we arrived, I found Mom to be fairly incoherent and unable to walk without assistance. I sat down beside her on the couch in the common area. She looked at me and began to describe what she was seeing. "Do you see that red house moving around over there?" pointing across the room. She spoke of seeing my father across the room, when he was actually sitting beside her. She began reading me words she was seeing on "big sheets of paper."

"Can't you see those words over there?" she urged.

"No, I can't see any words."

She looked at me, and said in a demanding voice, "Well, go get your glasses, so you can see!"

"Mom, I don't wear glasses."

She commented to me, "Well, you need some, so you can see better!"

The tears collected behind my eyelids several times during the visit as I sat beside her, listening to her talk nonsense, letting her describe the fantastical images playing out before her eyes. It was both painful and sad for me, and my stomach was tied up in knots. I felt physically ill. It was shocking to see so much deterioration in such a short time. Even more bizarre was her ability to retrieve all the necessary words to describe the fantastical images before her, yet her inability to call upon that same word retrieval to describe the present—the "reality" in which she actually existed.

As we sat together waiting for the holiday party to begin, she also repeated a version of something I'm told she'd been saying for the past few days to the caregivers. "Your dad doesn't need me anymore, and I just want to die now." I didn't know what to say in response, so I said nothing.

When mealtime arrived, she was nearly unable to walk to the table. It appeared her brain and her legs weren't communicating. Finally, with my assistance, we shuffled over to the buffet.

My mind was racing. *Did the unfortunate "medication mishap" cause this precipitous decline? Or, was this behavior a reaction to stopping her Alzheimer's medications a week ago? Could it happen that quickly? Was it, as Lionel believed, a series of small strokes robbing her of the ability to communicate clearly or walk steadily? How was she able to describe her hallucinations so clearly? Or was it as the Hospice nurse suggested, simply the normal progression of someone with severe Alzheimer's disease? Does anyone know? Why am I obsessing about this?* These questions circulated in my head as I sat down at the table with Lionel and my parents and attempted

223

to calm my anxiety enough to eat some of the holiday meal. My mother actually made an effort to eat, and Dad, seemingly unaffected by her bizarre behavior, was in the process of eating his usual healthy portion.

As I was attempting to force myself to eat, my cell phone rang. It was Dr. Nielson.

"Dr. Nielson, thank you so much for returning my call!" I stepped away from the dining table, and explained once more what had happened with Mom's medication.

Dr. Nielson responded with a heated, "What? That is completely unacceptable! She should have *never* been put back on the full dosage after being off of it for a week. The meds should have been restarted at a much smaller dose. It is no wonder she is having side effects! I will send an order to the facility to immediately stop the medication, and send a prescription for an entirely different drug for Sundowner's."

This was a clear case of too many fingers in the pie, exacerbated by poor lines of communication. How can things like this be avoided? I somehow restrained myself from calling the pharmacy used by Tendercare Cottages and melting down. And, not that I wanted to question the primary care physician's orders, but knowing now that there can be such intense side effects to restarting this type of medication at full strength, I wondered why he would do this.

Back at the table after this phone call, I began to experience feelings of relief that Dr. Nielson had a tangible plan to help Mom, so I relaxed and watched as my father finished his meal. By 6:30 p.m., Mom was ready to go to bed, so Lionel and I helped her to her room and the attendant came to help put on her pajamas. Emotionally depleted, I left the facility with Lionel shortly thereafter.

What would happen next? Thoughts of her bouncing back and regaining her appetite, along with ending Hospice care, danced through my mind. I wondered if this was some sort of undying optimism on my part, or if it was purely irrational thinking, or denial misguided by my hope to spend more time with my mom, even if she wasn't really the mom I used to know.

In the middle of the night, I awoke suddenly from a deep sleep with the realization that I had received another three-month supply of the Sundowner's medication in the mail a few days ago. It was currently sitting on my kitchen counter. Now that Dr. Nielson had switched medications, my mom was left with a four-month supply of a useless, expensive prescription drug. Tossing and turning in the darkness, I obsessed about this, feeling like I was wasting my parent's money, even though it was a completely unintentional consequence of an uncontrollable situation.

As I lay awake, alone with my thoughts, my brain moved on to other worries. I began to ruminate about Mom dying. Even though I believed I was prepared for this eventuality, every time I thought about it, I recognized this little pocket of anxiety, or maybe even despair, inside of me that I dared not touch because I sensed a grieving I couldn't yet bear to face. Maybe I wasn't as prepared as I thought. Was it just me, or was anyone ever really prepared?

My mother had not been *my mother* in more than three years. It was almost as if someone else inhabited her physical body. There had been a few times over the past couple years when she was suddenly present, like that afternoon I spent sewing buttons on her blouses, that I now cherished. Granted, the moments I could connect the mother of my childhood to the mother now in front of me were few and far between, but in those fleeting special moments there remained a safety, a security of *my mother* being close to me. I thought letting her go would be a relief, but I found there was an entire convoluted spectrum of emotions involved. These emotions were mixed and varied, a polarized balance of relief mixed with dread. There would be the relief of not watching her suffer with life, but it would also be a "letting go" of my *mama* who had known me since birth. The person who birthed me, and had known me for so long, and in such a different way than anyone else on this earth, would no longer live in this realm. I would join the ranks of so many others who have made this life transition. What would that be like? Was I ready to travel that path? Since I obviously had no choice in the matter, I was doing my best to prepare for the journey.

I looked at the clock, groaning with awareness that I had now been lying awake for well over an hour. I rolled over in bed and my thoughts turned to my father. For the past several years, I had been certain Dad would pass away first, given his advanced age and history of falls/broken bones. In fact, Mom and I were both certain Dad would pass away first. That's why we selected his burial outfit, and discussed the funeral three years ago. Now it's as if the reality of three years ago had turned on its head.

Before drifting off to sleep just before sunrise, I considered what someone had recently suggested to me—that my visits with my parents were more for me than them, and realized I disagreed. My visits were for all three of us. I believed that my parents were happy to have some companionship, even if they didn't always know me. Although we weren't usually having much of a conversation and my visits were most likely forgotten as soon as I left, while I was there it appeared to be meaningful to them, regardless of the level of depth or the plane of existence they were on. The concept of time was simply different for my parents.

During this time, I had difficulty coping with what felt like too many people involved in Mom's care. Tendercare Cottages had a rotation of different caregivers for every shift, some who kept better records than others, so no one was ever completely sure of Mom's chart's accuracy. When I called to ask how Mom was reacting to the new Sundowner's medication, there was no written record of her even having received it, even though the house administrator assured me she had been taking it for the past three days. Tendercare Cottages had Shelly, the staff nurse, who did her best to keep an eye on things, but because she traveled between five different facilities in three different towns, she was only at Tendercare Cottages a couple of times per week. She deferred to the Hospice nurse, Linda, who came once a week to do an assessment of Mom's condition. To top it off, it appeared that Mom's primary care doctor and psychiatrist didn't communicate with each other based on the incident with the paranoia/Sundowner's medication. There was also the pharmacy, which forgot I was in charge of ordering her medications. With this many people involved and the apparent lack of communication between them, it is no wonder that Mom's care sometimes seemed haphazard.

I often wished there was a central coordinator of care instead of all these individual pieces. I would have gladly volunteered for the position, but wondered how successful I would have been at getting the various people involved to regularly report back to me. It appeared the left hand didn't know what the right hand was doing with respect to my mother's care.

Lessons Learned

There needs to be open communication between you, the facility, the pharmacy (if applicable), and any of your loved one's physicians/mental health professionals. It would be prudent to have notes attached to the medication sheet for your loved one at both the pharmacy and the facility stating that if a medication runs out, to call you (in addition to the physician who *originally* prescribed the med). Granted, no plan is foolproof, but this may give you a chance to stay on top of the medications and prevent a serious mishap like the one that happened to Mom. It can be frustrating when you feel like there are too many people involved in the care of your loved one, or that all the caregivers/physicians involved are not communicating with each other, or with you. Remember that the facility caregivers and the physicians are doing their best to care for your loved one, and try to go with the flow and accept things as they come your way. If you are able, try to dialogue regularly with all caregivers involved in the care of your loved one so that you are aware of any new developments and/or miscommunication between the parties. Hopefully, you will be able to avoid any major mishaps. Realize, however, that this can be a time-consuming and exhausting role to play.

Remember that it's possible your loved one will get worse, then better, then worse again many times. Be prepared for this roller coaster, and do your best to ride the emotional ups and downs of dying. Seek out emotional support from a family member, friend, or support group.

THIRTY-NINE
Confusion, Expectations, and Theories

A few days after the holiday party, Mom strolled into the dining room for breakfast without wearing any pants. When the caregiver told her she had to put on her pants, she argued, "Well, I already have on pants!" Technically she was correct, in that she was wearing underpants, but nothing else besides her shirt and tennis shoes.

Shelly called and shared that story with me before saying, "I wanted to let you know I called and reported to Dr. Nielson that your mom continues to have behavior problems with wakefulness and restlessness at night, along with general confusion and unpredictable falls. I had a hunch she might possibly have a urinary tract infection, and the doctor agreed with me and ordered a urinalysis. We got the results back, and she has what we call around here a 'raging' UTI. This also provides yet another possible cause for her erratic behavior."

"Oh dear! I don't understand. Wouldn't she be complaining of pain? I've had a UTI and it hurts horribly! Why would you think she had a urinary tract infection?" I questioned. I silently wondered why they chose to call her psychiatrist about this rather than her primary care doctor.

"Well, amazingly, elderly people often don't feel any pain when they have a UTI. But all the other symptoms she's manifesting *are* often indicative of a urinary tract infection, so that's why I decided to call Dr. Nielson."

"How long do you think she's had it?" I inquired.

"We have no way of knowing that, unfortunately ... " her voice trailed off.

"I feel badly thinking that she has been suffering and we didn't realize sooner … "

"Vicki, I really don't think she's been in any pain, so please don't feel guilty. I wanted to ask how you felt about treating the infection with antibiotics, since she is in Hospice and you have requested palliative care only. How would you like to proceed?" she asked me.

"I'd like to treat the UTI with antibiotics. If there's even the slightest chance she may be experiencing pain, I want her to be comfortable. For me, the treatment falls under the banner of palliative care. Besides that, it has the potential to improve her quality of life," I reasoned.

High expectations are always dangerous, and things didn't go the way I expected. It took five days following the diagnosis of Mom's urinary tract infection for the antibiotics to appear at the facility, which was five days longer than I had hoped. Why did it take so long? No one was able to give me an answer.

It had now been eight days since the diagnosis when I made a late afternoon call to the facility to check up on her progress.

"Hi, how is my mom doing today?"

"Well, she fell out of bed again last night," replied Pat, the caregiver, "but didn't hurt herself. She's spent much of the afternoon reading an invisible book out loud. As usual, she hasn't eaten much of anything. And, oh yeah, we weighed her this morning, and she's lost another six pounds. I wish we could get her to eat something once in awhile, but she flatly refuses."

The antibiotics hadn't made a difference yet in diminishing her confusion and hallucinations, or helping her regain an appetite. Maybe in a few more days things would improve.

Pat also let me know the open sores (bedsores) on Mom's buttocks that she'd developed in the past couple of weeks were not getting better, but were, in fact, getting worse. These pressure sores were a chafing of the skin which occurred from sustained pressure cutting off the circulation to a "vulnerable" body part. This can happen in people who are sedentary, or have limited mobility caused by extensive sitting or being bedridden. Bedsores could also be caused by inadequate nutrition, which certainly applied to Mom. I hoped the Hospice nurse would be there tomorrow to check it out. My priority was to make my mother comfortable, and ease her pain however possible.

In trying to pinpoint a cause for Mom's behavior, we first blamed the abrupt stopping of the paranoia/Sundowner's Effect medication, and then the undiagnosed UTI. Lionel's hypothesis that she might be suffering a series of small strokes was also on my mind, especially thinking back to times in the distant past, several years ago, when I wondered if she might be having little mini strokes. At that time, she described a dizziness that lasted several minutes. Mini strokes could be responsible for the "incidents" she had had when she became unresponsive, and they could also be the cause of her continued confusion and seemingly accelerated brain disintegration, loss of verbal skills, and coordination.

I was now convinced this theory was a real possibility, especially in light of the physician's diagnosis of vascular dementia when she spent those two days in the hospital following her first major incident of unresponsiveness. At the time, I don't think I really processed this diagnosis because of my shock and worry about what was happening to her. I had since learned that vascular dementia occurred from a build-up of fat deposits in the artery walls (hardening of the arteries, called atherosclerosis), resulting in restricted blood flow to the brain, which could lead to strokes. The initial strokes from vascular dementia may be very minor (akin to the short dizzy spells Mom experienced and described to me a few years ago), and the symptoms may not be apparent until the mid-to-late stages of vascular dementia. Once vascular dementia progresses to the late stage, there can be a sudden, very noticeable decline in mental cognition and/or physical health in the person suffering from it, rather than the slower yet steady decline often associated with Alzheimer's disease.

While Mom didn't have a history of heart disease, hypertension, or diabetes (all telltale risk factors for developing vascular dementia), she did fit into the other two risk-factor categories of advanced age and smoking/passive smoking. "Closet smoker" best described my mother, who smoked for more than 50 years without her grandchildren ever knowing. She quit sometime in her seventies. She also had a family history of atherosclerosis, as her father was diagnosed with and died from hardening of the arteries in the early 1960s.

The type of vascular dementia that most accurately described my mother's symptoms/behavior is called "Multi-Infarct Dementia" (MID).[6] MID is caused by multiple strokes, where blood clots form in the brain, resulting in subsequent brain tissue death (see Appendix B)[2]. Motor and cognitive impairment, inappropriate social behavior, memory loss, confusion at night, depression, incontinence, delusions, and hallucinations are all symptomatic characteristics of MID,[7] and all appropriately described my mother's recent behavior.

Some research states that MID might, in fact, be a cause for Alzheimer's, or at least cause Alzheimer's to worsen at a quicker rate. While MID is often found in conjunction with Alzheimer's disease and is called "mixed dementia," it is also possible to misdiagnose MID as Alzheimer's disease, as many of the symptoms are the same.[8]

Did Mom have Alzheimer's disease, Multi-Infarct Dementia, or mixed dementia? This would always be an unanswered question for me, because I doubted there would be an autopsy performed when Mom passed. This new knowledge about Multi-Infarct Dementia did, however, provide another possible reason for her precipitous decline. I wondered if Alzheimer's disease had become something of a "catch-all" diagnosis for labeling people who display the symptoms associated with moderate-to-severe dementia simply because the medical community does not yet have a full understanding of this devastating disease. Whatever the cause, I knew that my mother's health and behavior had taken a turn for the worse.

[6] The obstruction of blood flow associated with vascular dementia is called infarction. Infarction involves the death of localized tissues caused by the blocking of the blood supply, usually by a blood clot or fragment of tissue. (Source: *Vascular Diseases and Vascular Dementia.* www.tree.com/health/dementia-causes-vascular.aspx).

[7] Hale, K. L. & Frank, J. (2005). *Dementia overview.* eMedicine Consumer Health.

Beers, M.H. & Berkow, R. (ed). (1999). *Dementia. The Merck Manual of Diagnosis and Therapy, 17th Edition.* Merck Research Laboratories, NJ, 1999.

[8]Jellinger, K.A. (2008). Morphologic diagnosis of "vascular dementia"-a critical update. *Journal of Neurological Science, 270*(1-2), 1-12. [Medline].

Jellinger, K.A. (2008). The pathology of "vascular dementia": a critical update. *Journal of Alzheimer's Disease, 14*(1), 107-123. [Medline].

FORTY
Restlessness

When I called to check on Mom yesterday evening, she had been taking the antibiotics for her UTI for five days. My call was answered after only a few rings. "Oh, hi Vicki, this is Jody. I was just looking up your phone number to call and let you know your mom's fallen again, but seems to be okay. She's taken up a kind of ceaseless pacing back and forth, back and forth, the past few nights. We're still having a lot of trouble getting her to bed, let alone keeping her there. We've had to start locking your dad's door because she keeps going in there and waking and disturbing him in the middle of the night."

"Oh," I sighed, "poor Dad. And, I was so hoping to hear the antibiotics might be helping the falling and restlessness by now…you're sure she's okay? No obvious bruises or bumps?"

"No, she appears to be completely fine. Maybe we'll notice some improvement with the restlessness after she's been on the antibiotics a few more days. Last night, I convinced her to sit in her recliner for a few minutes while I was charting in the main room. Suddenly I heard a loud thud and when I ran into her room, there she was, lying face down on the floor! She'd fallen out of the recliner and was sprawled out on the carpet, surrounded by a pool of water spilling out from her upturned water bottle."

"I often wonder how many more times she can fall before she does hurt herself. I wish there was something we might do to protect her, but I don't know what it is."

"I don't know either," Jody sighed, "but she's been lucky so far, hasn't she? We really do our best to keep a close eye on her. We've begun to notice in the past few days she's stopped using her walker. It's almost like she has no clue what it's for, so it sits unused in a corner of her room. For that matter, I don't think she really understands what to do with food, either. Yesterday we caught her just in the nick of time, as she was getting ready to dump a bowl of soup into her lap. She plays with her food, tips over liquids, and even managed to pull her neighbor's placemat onto the floor, scattering silverware all over the hardwood floor. She no longer seems to have any interest in eating food, only in playing with it."

"It sounds like having a mischievous little kid in the house," I responded sadly.

"She keeps us all on our toes, that's for sure. Oh, I almost forgot to tell you one other thing. You'll be pleased to hear that Linda from Hospice stopped by today and tended to the sores on your mom's bum. They're already looking a little better."

"Well, it's good to hear at least one bit of good news!" I exclaimed. "I'll be out tomorrow to visit. Is there anything either of them need?"

"Not that I can think of. If something comes to mind, though, I'll call you back. Well, I'd better get back to my charting."

"Okay, thanks for the update."

"You bet. Take care!"

FORTY-ONE
Rubber Ball

Today was a difficult day. Listening to the caregivers' description of Mom's behavior over the phone and actually witnessing it were two different things. I thought I was prepared.

I wasn't.

When I arrived, Mom was attempting to push Dad's wheelchair. They appeared to be going *some*where, but only she knew where. She looked up, saw me, and smiled. I could see a flash of obvious recognition.

"Hi," I greeted them and offered to push Dad's chair, so she could push her walker, and we could "walk" together. The staff was right. It appeared she *couldn't* figure out how to push the walker. She was frozen to the spot where she stood. While I attempted to wheel Dad by, she scolded, "Stop it!" but it was not clear what she meant.

While I was trying to help her with the walker, Dad, looking straight ahead, wheeled himself past Mom and me over to the dining room table. I decided it might be easier for her to take my arm, and together we could walk to the table, but she didn't want to do that. She was rooted in place; it was as if she had momentarily forgotten how to make her legs move. I wasn't sure what to try next.

At that moment, Sally, the Hospice social worker, arrived for a visit. With the two of us each holding an arm, we convinced those legs of Mom's to move forward, but only after considerable effort and encouragement. Eventually, we seated her at the table next to Dad, and the four of us proceeded to have a conversation.

To date, this was the most bizarre, illogical conversation I had ever had. Mom was particularly chatty. She would say several coherent words, and then suddenly tumble into nonsense words, so a clear thought never actually made it out of her mouth. Her speech pattern was reminiscent of Helen, the woman at Cedar Grove who had called me "skurpy." Sally, an experienced medical social worker, was adept at asking questions and interpreting what Mom was attempting to say, which to me sounded completely unintelligible. I tried to listen closely and pick up clues about what Mom was trying to communicate.

"Tell Louise that she can come spankles if she darbies, but I have to pluck the beans before sklosh dopens plune." *Perhaps she was talking about Louise, her friend growing up.*

"Oh Buster, please can I go ice skating with you? The steak is ready right now and you sculp mantens spooch!" *She must be talking to the neighbor who lived on the nearby farm when she was a child.* Apparently she was reliving the past, albeit in some other dimension.

When she started talking about "boiling babies," however, it was increasingly difficult to stay in the conversation. It was mentally challenging, especially given the nonsensical gibberish I was trying to understand. I was concentrating very hard, attempting to make some sense—any sense—out of what she was saying. She was trying so hard to complete sentences. At the end of this conversation, I believed we were all drained of energy in our attempts to link two separate universes.

Mom was able to clearly convey one phrase: "We need to leave now," which she repeated numerous times that afternoon, always followed by an attempt to stand up and walk away. Each time, I stopped her from standing by placing some pressure on her thighs with my hands, and directly asking her a question of some sort to distract her. She seemed restless, and when she decided to stand up yet again, Sally and I watched, seemingly paralyzed as the scene went into slow motion, and Mom began moving away from the table. It was as if we were frozen to our chairs, helplessly watching as she began swaying back and forth, back and forth. Suddenly the spell was broken, and we leapt out of our chairs, but not fast enough. Everyone nearby tried unsuccessfully to reach her as she teetered precariously, and then toppled over backwards, landing flat on her back on the hardwood floor. All of us watched aghast as her head hit the floor with a deafening thud. Then, unexpectedly, she bounced back up, just like a rubber ball! She stood up and looked at us, seemingly unscathed by her fall, and within a few moments, had no memory of falling.

We helped her sit back down, and Sally checked her over to be sure she was all right. Sally looked at me and ventured, "I believe your mom might be safer in a wheelchair with a seat belt." After witnessing this disturbing scene, I was in full agreement. Mom was shaky and unsteady, and so terribly confused.

Keeping her seated for the rest of the afternoon was a challenge. About the only thing that kept her relaxed and sitting still in her chair was a continuous neck and shoulder massage. As we sat together, she was also doing some imaginary sewing, right down to the threading of a needle. She made continuous picking motions at her pants, as if she were snatching lint, a common trait of someone with Alzheimer's disease.

Pat came over to the table where the four of us were seated. "Vicki, despite that fall a few minutes ago, I think your mom's doing much better today than even three days ago, when she was acting like a zombie all day. We got rid of the box springs and let her sleep on just the mattress on the floor last night. She stayed in bed!"

"Getting rid of the box springs sounds like a very sensible solution. I know I will rest easier knowing if she falls out of bed, she won't be falling very far!"

"One other thing I wanted to tell you is that tomorrow Linda will be here to retest her to see if the UTI's cleared up."

"I'm glad to hear that. I sure hope it's cleared up!"

In the end, it seemed we were still guessing what was causing Mom's latest behavior patterns, whether it was her medication, the UTI, or the natural progression of Alzheimer's (or MID), or perhaps a combination of all three. *Did the answer really even matter anymore?* The somber fact remained—overall she was exhibiting a massive decline in both physical and mental health.

FORTY-TWO
Prolonging Life

"Hi, Pat! How are things at Tendercare Cottages today?" I had stopped by to drop off some "Electric Shave" for the caregivers to use before they shaved Dad today. Yesterday I noticed the skin surrounding his mouth had a visibly sore, bright red appearance. He wasn't complaining, but it looked painful.

"It's a grand day at Tendercare!" laughed Pat. "Linda's here right now with your Mom," she said, tipping her head in the direction of Mom's closed door. "I'm sure it would be okay if you joined them."

I walked across the common area, past several residents watching *One Life to Live* on the TV, and knocked on Mom's door.

"Yes?" I could hear Linda's voice in response to my knock.

"Hi, Linda, it's me, Vicki."

"Oh hi, Vicki, come on in. I'm just finishing up your mom's assessment," she indicated as I strode into Mom's room.

"Hi, Mom. How are you doing today?" I looked over to where Mom was sitting on her mattress, babbling nonsensically. She didn't acknowledge me or look in my direction. I walked over, kneeled down, and gave her a gentle hug. As I sat down on the floor beside Mom, Linda joined us. "She seems to be in her own little world this afternoon, doesn't she?" she said.

I nodded, "Yeah, I wish I could understand what she's talking about."

"This isn't an easy time for you, is it, having to see your mom like this? You'll be glad to hear I rechecked her this afternoon and the UTI has cleared up."

That meant it was probably safe to rule out the UTI as a reason for her behavioral issues. The antibiotics had not proven to be a cure-all, after all.

"I *am* glad to hear that, of course, but had hoped it might have made a difference with her wakefulness and restlessness at night," I sighed disappointedly.

"Yes, that would have been a better outcome, wouldn't it? It appears the mattress on the floor *is* working to keep her from falling out of bed, but according to what Pat told me, your mom was up all night again, and just woke up shortly before I got here this afternoon. So yes, you are right, the antibiotics don't seem to have helped with that. She continues to amaze everyone with her energy level and stamina during the night!"

I, in contrast, was not surprised that she was still holding on with a ferocity that was inexplicable to most. I don't think they realized just how stubborn this woman had been her whole life.

Linda continued, "When I had her stand up a little while ago, she was pretty shaky, weak, and unsteady, probably partly from a lack of calories. She's lost more than five pounds since last week, dropping below 105."

I nodded in agreement; she was definitely looking thinner.

Linda went on, "Pat mentioned that she hand-fed her some canned pears at lunch today, and then coaxed her into drinking three quarters of a glass of Ensure, along with a cup of water."

I thought about this for a minute. Was I supposed to hail this as a victory? Slowly and carefully, I inquired, "I am wondering *why* they are having her drink the Ensure and hand-feeding her. Do you have any insight into this?"

Her answer was simple, "Well, basically it's to prolong her life."

This confirmed what I already knew, but wanted to hear someone else verbalize aloud. In my mind, this type of intervention did not coincide with Mom's end-of-life wishes described in both her living will and the *Comfort One* measure. This situation presented a dilemma for me. What was the right thing to do? Mom explicitly did not want any heroic measures prolonging the dying process. Should they continue to cajole, coax, and wheedle her into taking nourishment? Would doing anything less be inhumane? I wasn't sure. What would Mom say?

Knowing that this was a delicate subject, and not wanting to come across as uncaring, I hesitantly responded, "I thought that as part of her wishes for end-of-life care, she wanted to be comfortable, but not prolong the dying process. It seems to me she might consider being forced to eat not adhering with her wishes."

Linda replied, "You know, in my opinion that's the healthy attitude. Most people wish to keep their family member alive as long as possible, by whatever means necessary. It's almost as if they are blind to what their loved one is going through. The family members don't ask the question: *What is this person's quality of life?* Are we doing interventions to extend their life for *them* or for *ourselves*? You seem to have a very healthy relationship with the process of life and death. I'll speak to the caregivers again about your wishes, or I guess I should say your mother's wishes."

I looked at her with appreciation and thanked her. I was relieved that she seemed to understand what I was saying, and I didn't feel as if she was negatively judging me.

As my mother had wished, I had already requested care as described in *Comfort One,* but evidently, the staff was not adhering to it. I pondered that it was difficult for human beings to let go. How did we get to this place, where humans were kept alive with hand feeding, force-fed nutrition shakes, or worse, tubes for feeding or breathing?

I found I was much too tentative about saying anything to the caregivers, or anyone else for that matter, because I was afraid they would judge me and perceive me as uncaring. I had seen and read information on numerous occasions reporting that it was more the social "norm" in our culture to keep people with us in this world as long as possible, by whatever means deemed necessary. How often *did* people ask what the quality of life was when these decisions about prolonging life were made? I did care about not making this any more difficult for my mother *(and myself?)* than it already was. The truth was Mom was not going to get better. She was not going to regain her memory or vitality. I knew this in my heart as well as in my head. It wasn't as if I wanted her to die faster; I simply didn't wish to prolong her suffering.

As I sat there next to Mom, reflecting on these thoughts, the tears trickled down my face. I appreciated Linda's validation of my concerns and feelings, but it didn't make the futility of the situation any easier. I looked over at Mom, who was lying on the mattress, her frail body shaking and shivering, even though the room was very warm. Occasionally, she jabbered some gibberish, although it was unclear to me if she realized we were sitting beside her. I stroked her hair, and she seemed to visibly relax.

We sat in silence for a few moments and then, Linda said softly, "This is a difficult time for family—for you—and there are a lot of hard decisions to be made. It's never an easy process."

"How long do you foresee her going on like this?" I queried through my tears, not sure if she would even be able to address this question.

"Well, if her behavior and eating habits continue as they have, it's possible she'll survive for several months or more, provided she doesn't become ill."

I digested this information, which seemed quite plausible, even though it was hard to think of Mom continuing to suffer that long.

"Based on what happened yesterday when Sally was here, I also feel it would be a wise idea to order a wheelchair with a seat belt installed, so that she's less likely to fall and break a bone."

"Yes, I think that's probably sensible, but I wonder how she's going to accept being strapped in a wheelchair. I can only imagine how angry that will make her," I surmised with some hesitation.

"I think there's a good chance she may not even be aware of what's happening, given her present state. For her safety, would you consider at least trying it?"

We agreed to order the wheelchair with a seat belt.

Lesson Learned

If your loved one is in Hospice care and you are confused about what steps to take about your loved one's care, reach out to the Hospice team. Their advice, support, and validation helped me immensely. If your loved one is not in Hospice care and you need advice or support, try contacting a medical social worker experienced in dealing with end-of-life issues, as he or she may be a valuable source of information. Your local hospital or Alzheimer's Association should be able to connect you with a qualified professional.

FORTY-THREE
The Spitting Llama

It was two days before Christmas. Why was I so melancholy at this most joyous time of year? I didn't have to search very far or deep to find an answer: my mother's worsening condition. I realized that this was going to be the last Christmas she'd be with us. I'd learned there was no way a person could completely grieve ahead of time, even if one made an attempt to do so. Grieving had to occur in due course, at the proper time. Anticipatory grieving may help take the edge off, but the real and true grieving cannot be done ahead of time. I felt like I'd been grieving for more than three years, but the actuality of her passing within the next few months was now upon me, and this was a different, more vivid type of grieving. The person I could call for ideas whenever life threw a challenge my way had been gone a long time, and now the outside shell was also fading. This shell housed a most demented person, lost and alone in her own world. Talking with her reminded me of having a telephone conversation with a bad connection. Every few words were lost, and it was difficult to follow what she was attempting to say. I was overcome with feelings of frustration and helplessness.

"Hello? This is Vicki calling. How are my parents today?" It was mid-afternoon, and between wrapping presents and preparing dinner for my family, I called to check on Mom and Dad.

"Oh, hi Vicki. This is Karen. Your Dad's been wheeling around the facility all afternoon having a grand time. We have to keep an eye on him though, 'cause he likes to go in other resident's rooms and swipe things. Innocently enough, you understand. I think he's just bored. Right now he's in his room watching TV. Your mom's been sleeping most of the day. Pat and I were just talking about getting her up, seeing if she'd drink a little water and maybe join the other residents for our Christmas carol sing-a-long this afternoon."

"Oh, that's good. I was wondering if her wheelchair had arrived yet?"

"Yes, it did, shortly after you left a couple of days ago. We had quite a time with her in the beginning. When Pat and I sat her in it and buckled the seat belt, she started to fuss saying 'You can't do this to me.' I felt bad making her sit in it, but it's for her safety."

"Yes, of course, you're right. I'm sorry, too, that we have to confine her this way."

"What happened next would have been funny if it hadn't been so sad," continued Karen. "She wheeled herself around the common room acting like a llama and spitting at the other residents! After we explained about ten times that the chair was to keep her safe so she wouldn't fall and hurt herself, she seemed to catch on, at least on some level. She's been a little lamb about it ever since."

"Oh, thank you, Karen. I'm so glad you and Pat are there to take care of my parents. I hope she didn't upset the other residents too much."

"For what it's worth, I didn't notice any reaction from the other residents."

When I called the facility the next day, Pat informed me that Mom had been moved to the other dining table for meal-time where "messy eaters" were seated, due to complaints re-

ceived from others at her dining table about her "table man-
ners." Evidently, she was again seated for meals at the same
time as everyone else. At this new table, if she wanted to tip
over her juice and play with her food, no one would mind.
If she wanted to stack her scrambled eggs into a tower and
set her donut on top as if she were constructing architectural
masterpieces made from edible Legos, that was okay too.

Pat also shared that Mom was now zipping around the facility in her wheelchair as if she was a seasoned "driver," and
the chair her chariot. There had been no more complaints
from her about sitting in it.

FORTY-FOUR
"Who are you?"

There was little traffic on Christmas morning when Lionel and I drove across town to visit my parents. The sky was grey and everything was covered in a mantle of white from the previous night's snowfall. It was a classic white Christmas. As I opened the front door at Tendercare Cottages, the tinkling of the sleigh bells on the inside window was the only sound we heard. It was very quiet, with no one about except the two caregivers, who were sitting at the dining room table charting. From where we stood in the entryway, we were able to look into both of my parents' rooms and see their backs as they sat in their wheelchairs, each absorbed in their own world. We strode into their rooms and noted that Mom was awake, staring off into space, and Dad was sleeping. Even though I had described my mother's condition to Lionel, he was unprepared for the current reality. He had last seen Mom three weeks ago, and her abilities had declined drastically since then. Conversation was challenging, and Lionel experienced this first-hand today.

I attempted to awaken Dad, but he apparently wasn't in the mood to open his eyes. We pushed his wheelchair into Mom's room, and I knelt down beside her, looked up at her and said, "Hi." For the first time, zero recognition flashed in her eyes, and she said to me, "Who are you?" Even though I had been expecting this, my heart sank as I assimilated the fact that, at least for today, my mother no longer recognized me. I told her who I was and she stared at me blankly. As she sat slouched in her wheelchair, she looked down at her sunken stomach and remarked, "If this gets any fatter, they won't let me eat." We sat in silence for a few moments as I searched for something to say or do.

Noticing that Mom's Christmas present from the facility was stuffed into her opened dresser drawer, still wrapped, and seeing a potential avenue for interaction, I asked, "Mom, should we open your Christmas present and see what Santa brought you?"

She answered with an unenthusiastic, "Okay," and I sensed she had little interest in the whole event. Santa had brought her a new pair of jeans (but, why a size 16 for this tiny woman?) and some white socks.

A few minutes later, my brother Jack and his family called to say "Merry Christmas," and since Dad was still asleep, Jack attempted to talk to Mom.

"Hi, Mom. Merry Christmas."

"Who are you?"

"This is your son, Jack."

"Well, *that's* a new one!"

After a few more attempts at conversation, I heard an audible, "Well, take care, Mom."

Mom mumbled something unintelligible in response. I gently took the phone back from her.

Lionel and I sat with them for another hour or so before it was time for us to depart. I leaned over to give Mom a kiss and say goodbye, and she mumbled (to no one in particular), "I hate myself. I'm going to kill myself. Then you'll be sorry."

Wow. Where did that old memory come from? It didn't seem as though she were talking to me, thankfully! It must have come from somewhere out of her past. Off-hand, disturbing comments such as this left me thinking she still harbored some internal torment. I had long hoped she might at last experience inner peace, but it was not yet the case.

With a sigh and an errant tear, I wistfully said my good-bye to Mom and Dad, leaving them sitting side-by-side in their wheelchairs, chins resting on their chests, lost in the sleep of waiting on this silent Christmas morning.

Lesson learned

No matter how much you think you prepare yourself for the day when your loved one no longer recognizes you, it is still going to be difficult to accept. Unfortunately, it's likely that this will, at some point, occur. Reach out to others, whether it's friends, relatives, caregivers, or Hospice. Find someone with a listening ear, as it can help the grieving process to talk about these changes.

FORTY-FIVE
Fallen off the Cliff

Two days after Christmas, my son Kyle and his fiancé Kylee arrived for a few days, and I took them with me to Tendercare Cottages for an afternoon visit. No amount of prior warning could have prepared Kyle for what he was about to witness. Lionel had commented to Kyle and Kylee that Mom had "slipped," but after spending time with her today Kyle's response was "She's not simply slipped, she's fallen off the cliff entirely!"

The caregivers had gotten Mom out of bed a short time before we arrived mid-afternoon. Previous attempts to awaken her were met with resistance; she repeatedly told them she was "too tired to get up." She and Dad were sitting side-by-side in their wheelchairs in the dining area when we arrived. Mom was silently staring off into space, and Dad appeared to be asleep. The three of us walked over, pulled up some chairs and joined them. I introduced all of us, several times. Dad was sleepy for most of our visit, but Mom was in a conversational mood today. Not surprisingly, we couldn't understand most of what she was saying. Some words or sentences came out clearly, but made no real sense. Other sentences came out with garbled or made-up words, which made it even more challenging to carry on a conversation with her. There was a lot of head nodding in agreement with whatever she was trying to say, unless her body language indicated we should be expressing concern and/or not smiling. This was a guessing game, and took a bit of improvisational acting.

One sentence came out clearly: "I'm starving."

Pat, who heard Mom say this, looked to me for permission before making her some toast. As I had feared, my "wishes" that I had discussed earlier with Linda concerning not unnecessarily prolonging Mom's life had been misinterpreted by the Tendercare Cottages staff members; it was apparent by the look on Pat's face that she was afraid I would be upset if she gave Mom something to eat. *What kind of horrible daughter-monster do they think I am?*

"Please, if she asks for food, let her have *whatever* she wants to eat," I assured Pat. "My only request is that you don't force her to eat by hand-feeding her food when she blatantly doesn't want it." *How could I make them understand this?* Pat made Mom a piece of toast, which she ate and then washed down with some white grape juice, surprising us all. Noticing my surprise, Pat told me that Mom had been eating lately, but very small portions.

Overall, Mom was acting less agitated. She was in high spirits this afternoon, and smiled and giggled as we "visited." Once she did scold Dad about something he had done (which was unclear), and he simply nodded his head in tacit agreement, even though he probably had no idea what she was chastising him about. She then looked right at us and clearly stated, "Your Dad was walking," paused for a moment and then looked at Dad and said, "Isn't that right? You were walking?" Without missing a beat, he agreed with her that he had been walking. I'm not sure if he believed it himself or was just agreeing to stay out of trouble with her. This type of response by my dad had a very long history. Not wanting to provoke her wrath, he was often known to agree with her, even when she was obviously incorrect.

At one point during the visit, Dad grabbed her hand and said, "Good night! Your hands are like ice!" We smiled at this outburst, which was one of the only times he spoke while we were there. At that particular moment, they looked so endearing sitting together with him holding her cold hand. I was glad they had each other, even if sometimes they didn't know who the other was; strangers or not, they seemed to be comforted by one another's presence. Today Mom was like a marshmallow; her brittleness had disappeared, exposing a softened, pliant exterior. Life appeared to have calmed to a place where both Mom and Dad were relaxed while awaiting their departure from this life.

Dad seemed to grow bored with our company and rolled off in his wheelchair in the direction of his room. Kyle and Kylee decided to follow him while I stayed at the table beside Mom. Shelly, the facility nurse, stopped by to chat with me for a moment and shared, "I feel there's been definite improvement in your mother's condition over this last week, as far as her eating is concerned. She's been eating up to 80 percent of her meal." While heartening at first, I reminded myself that her portions were essentially tablespoon size.

Shelly also commented, "Also, her bedsores have almost healed!" She then paused for a moment before continuing, "That's the good news. On the not-so-positive side, she's lost another couple of pounds. At night, the staff continues to find her walking around her room naked. They do their best to keep tabs on her, but sometimes they're attending to other residents."

"Yeah, I understand. It's not like we can tie her to her bed or make her sleep in her wheelchair … "

"No, of course not. It's a dilemma and a challenge, but I have to say, I think the staff here does a good job for the most part."

"Well, no one can watch her 24/7 and I agree, I believe they do a good job too. They treat the residents well. It's just so sad to helplessly watch the rapid decline, feeling like there's nothing I can do to ease the way for her."

"Ah, but you are already doing it, Vicki! You are *here* for her ... your love and commitment to her is quite apparent."

I reflected on this comment as Kyle, Kylee, and I gathered our coats, hats and gloves. Goodbye hugs were given, and we were on our way. The air felt frigid, and the snow crunched underfoot as we walked toward my car in the late afternoon. Sunlight was waning and the temperature biting, but my heart felt warm with Shelly's words.

FORTY-SIX
Spitfire

It was January 1, 2008. I sat at my kitchen counter with my morning cup of tea, and reflected on how different this year would undoubtedly be. Somberly, I realized this would most likely be Mom's last year with us. There was nothing to be done to change that outcome. My New Year's resolution would be to attempt to maintain a sense of equanimity throughout the progression of Mom's final journey.

Linda had done her weekly assessment of Mom yesterday and called me afterwards. "The staff tells me your mom's still up wandering around half the night. No one knows where she gets the energy, but it's a concern that she's still so restless. Her weight's dropped below 100 pounds, although she continues to eat minute amounts. We've run into a problem with her morning pill regimen. When the staff attempts to administer them, she just spits the pills back out. They've tried crushing them and mixing them into her pudding, and she still spits them back out, along with the food."

My mind wandered as she spoke. *Why did this remind me of a time when our family dog took medication and we rolled the pill inside cheese hoping to trick our dog into taking his pill, but he always managed to eat the cheese and spit the pill back out?*

My attention bounced back to the conversation when Linda said, "The facility's asked my permission to stop some of your mother's pills, like the antacid, the pain medication for her arthritis, and her antidepressant. How do you feel about discontinuing them?"

"Well ..." I chose my words carefully, "it's my impression that the antacid isn't doing anything to help encourage her appetite, so I have no problem stopping that. Since she spends most of her time in the wheelchair, I think it's probably okay to stop the pain medication for her arthritis. Obviously, if she begins to complain about knee pain, that's another story." I paused to consider the antidepressant. "Do you think the antidepressant could still be helping with her mood?"

"That's certainly possible, so maybe we could continue that pill, but move it to the evening, to be taken along with her Sundowner's medication. At least for now, she doesn't seem to mind taking pills at night. We'll continue to re-evaluate this as time goes on," she added.

"Hi, this is Vicki calling. I wanted to wish everyone at Tendercare a Happy New Year and ask how Mom is feeling today."

"Hi Vicki, Pat here. Thank you and Happy New Year to you too! Your mom's been quiet today. Probably because she gave us such a hard time last night ... she did NOT want to stay in her bed. It's amazing to all of us because she hasn't really eaten or drunk anything for a couple of days, but still somehow has the energy to act out!"

"This really concerns me," I began. "Both Shelly and the Hospice nurse told me that Mom's still getting up and wandering around at night. I'm afraid she's going to fall and break her hip or something. Since I talked to them, I've been thinking about what we might do to keep her safe. I was wondering if we could possibly attach some sort of tab alarm, like my father has, to her pajamas that would alert you if she tried to stand up?"

"Well, that might work if she'd leave her pajamas on!" Pat responded. "Actually, last night was different because she *wasn't* standing and walking. She was *crawling* around on the floor. She also prefers sleeping right on the floor instead of on her mattress."

I parroted Pat's information, "Let's see … not only is she still taking off her pajamas, but now she's sleeping on the carpet when she's not off crawling around somewhere? Oh my goodness." I digested that for a few seconds before suggesting, "If that's the case, is it possible you might put down a mat beside her mattress on the floor?" thinking that was preferable to the scratchy institutional carpeting.

"You know, that's a good idea. I'll see if I can find some sort of soft pad to set beside her mattress. She's easy to care for during the day because she sleeps so much. We just know we have to keep a closer eye on her at night. There's no doubt in our minds that your Mom's just a little spitfire who can still cause quite a ruckus around here."

"Who knows? Maybe she has a secret stash of food in her room giving her all that night energy," I joked.

Pat chuckled, "Yeah, who knows?"

"What's Dad been doing today?" I changed the subject.

"Oh, your dad's had a good day. He's rung in the New Year with a little paper-horn noisemaker. He spent a good part of the morning rolling around the building blowing his horn. Right now he's sitting in the common area with some of the other residents, still wearing his Happy New Year hat."

FORTY-SEVEN
Just Scooting Along

"Hi, I was calling to see if Mom was awake before I came to visit." It was three days into the New Year.

"Well, your mom got a shower this morning," said Pat, not directly answering my question, "and then we took her over to the other building's beauty shop to have her hair shampooed and set. She just came back a few minutes ago and said she's exhausted, so we put her to bed for a nap on her new double bed."

"Her new double bed?" I inquired.

"Yes! We think we've found a solution to her getting out of bed at night. We took away the box springs and put two single mattresses together on the floor, kind of like a king-sized bed. She has more room to move around and hasn't fallen or crawled out of bed for the last two nights."

I waited until later in the afternoon to visit, giving Mom time for her nap. When I arrived, her bedroom door was closed. I cracked it open and peeked into the darkened room. She was all curled up in a ball on her mattress on the floor, sound asleep. As I stood in the doorway staring at my Mom, such a tiny, frail being, tears leaked out the corners of my eyes. I wasn't ready to face what I was seeing quite yet, so I softly closed the door. I decided to go say hello to Dad and collect my emotions. Sometimes denial was my coping mechanism.

Dad was scooting down the hallway in his wheelchair. "Where are you headed?" I asked him.

"I don't know. Somewhere that's good. Where would you suggest?"

I had long since learned that it can be extremely disorienting and agitating to a dementia patient to continually bring them back to reality, so I thought I'd indulge him with a little fantasy. "How about Hawaii?" I ventured.

He replied, "That sounds good, but first I have to go potty," so off I went to find someone to help him.

While he was busy, I walked over to talk to Shelly, who was charting in the office.

"Oh, hi Vicki. I was actually just charting on your mom. Now that we've put your mom's mattresses on the floor, her headboard's been just leaning up against the wall. Hospice has asked the facility to remove it, along with her nightstand, because they consider them hazardous when your mom's moving around so much at night. If you want, we can store the furniture in the spare room where we put her box springs, until you can decide what to do with them."

I heaved a big sigh, "Thank you for offering to store them. I really appreciate the offer, and I agree. It's a good idea to move the furniture out of there." We were slowly deconstructing her room while her body was slowly deconstructing itself.

Fresh tears began to seep out of my eyes as Shelly began to talk about Mom's current condition. "She's not been interested in eating or drinking anything today, nor has she had much for the past several days. We're watching her grow visibly weaker, although amazingly, she somehow continues to have energy in the evenings. We're still able to give her the two remaining meds, crushed up and mixed into a little bit of pudding. This has pretty much been her sole source of calories lately."

I acknowledged the information with a nod. I couldn't think of anything to say to such news. "Do you think it would be okay to wake her up now?" I asked.

"Yes, that's a good idea. I'll come with you," and we walked through the dining area to Mom's room.

I kneeled on the floor beside her mattresses, lightly touched her shoulder and called her name. She immediately began mumbling very softly and unintelligibly as I said, "Hi, Mom. It's Vicki, here to see you." I held her cold hand while the nurse checked her heart.

"Her heart is slowing down. Note how her skin stays tented when I pull and pinch it slightly. That's a sign of dehydration. You can see the coloring in her feet is still fine, though. At the end of life, circulation often slows down so much that the feet take on a bluish hue. I have to say, this is the worst I've seen her," Shelly added gravely.

Suddenly, in a clear voice, Mom said, "I want to go home now." Perhaps that had a double meaning?

Shelly left us then and I parked myself beside Mom on the mattress, stroking her head and praying as the tears spilled down my cheeks. "Oh, God, please be merciful and take my mother home. Please, please let her fall asleep one more time, and take her on that final journey." Over and over I silently repeated this emotional prayer as I stroked her cheek or head and held her hand. Suddenly, she coughed like she was choking and for a split second I thought, *Oh no, this is happening right now*, realizing even though I was praying for her release from this life, I was still unprepared for that inevitable moment. But no, she was only coughing. I sighed with relief. I looked closely at her and a tear rolled out of her eye. Was it from coughing or something else? *What world was she in right now?*

She slept on as I remained beside her on the mattress. It reminded me of watching my children sleep when they were tiny, new infants recently home from the hospital. As a new, fearful mother, I watched to be sure they were still breathing. This was what I was doing as I sat beside Mom, except this time I was a fearful daughter, watching for the steady rise and fall of her chest as she breathed in and out, in and out. Emotionally depleted, and with her sleeping peacefully, I left her room to spend some time with Dad.

"What are you up to, Dad?" I asked him, to which he replied, "Getting ready to go to bed."

"Will you have supper first?"

He answered, "Yes," and put his chin back on his chest to catch another "40 winks" before supper. I patted him on the back of his head and gave him a swift kiss on the cheek.

I walked back into Mom's room and looked around. I decided to bring home what was left of my mother's costume jewelry along with a large, white ceramic cat, several knick-knacks, and her phone and clock. It seemed appropriate to remove some of the more tangibly memorable keepsakes, as well as items she no longer needed. My stomach felt knotted as I filled the backseat of my car with part of my mother's life. Would the grieving ever end?

I called the facility later in the evening. "Hello. This is Vicki. Did Mom eventually wake up?"

"Hi Vicki," said Jody, "Yes, she got up around 7 p.m. and said, 'I am damn dry.' She then proceeded to drink nearly 24 ounces of water and sip part of a bowl of tomato soup. You know what this means, don't you?"

"Um, that she won't want to go back to bed tonight?"

"I wouldn't think so, after sleeping most of the day. Guess what she's doing at the moment?"

"Crawling around her bedroom floor?" I asked.

"Yep. She's scooting around her room on her bottom having a good time, with intermittent stops to stare at her wall. I'll have time to spend with her after we get the rest of the residents to bed."

"Oh, thank you. I'm so glad to know you are there for her, and that she's safe. I'll talk to you later," I said as we ended our conversation.

It was 4:30 a.m. and I was awake perseverating over my latest dilemma, which involved my family and travel. Many months ago, my two older children and their significant others, along with Lionel and I, arranged a trip to visit my youngest daughter Jill, who lived in Egypt. We planned to be gone for two weeks, leaving at the end of January, which was now only a couple of weeks away. I had mixed emotions as the trip drew near. *Should I be leaving the country at a time like this? What if she passed away while I was out of town?* Everyone around me told me to go, including the Hospice caregivers, the facility caregivers, my friends, relatives, and co-workers. I knew Mom would have said the same thing, but somehow it seemed callous to think of leaving. Was I merely attempting to justify my actions by saying Mom would have told me to go? Honestly, I thought not; Mom would have said something she often said to me before the disease convinced her I was using her money for these trips: "Go! Life is for the living." My introspections always brought me back to the same question. What was the right thing to do?

Lessons Learned

No matter how much you want to be at the side of your loved one for every up and down, try not to completely put your own life on hold, because ultimately you do not have control over the recovery or the decline of your loved one's health. Take my mother's advice: "life is for the living." As hard as it may be, you have to remember this and not be consumed by guilt over living *your* life. Working through the guilt is an important emotional process, and will ultimately help you reach a place of peace amidst the pain of this journey.

FORTY-EIGHT
A Surreal World

Ten days passed. I'd made a couple of visits during that time, and daily phone calls. The facility staff told me most days passed peacefully, although Mom's nights were often anxious and sometimes combative. Jody shared an example of this.

"A couple nights ago, when I checked on your mom around 10 o'clock, there she was, lying on her mattress with her legs and butt right up against the wall, feet pointing to the ceiling! I tried to coax her back on to her mattress, saying, 'Come on, honey, let's lay you back down,' but your mom started hollering, 'No, no, no!' and pushed me away. I called Karen to come in and help me, but your mom was acting pretty combative and completely stubborn, insisting on staying in that awkward position. I warned her, 'sweetie, your legs and feet are gonna go to sleep.' It took awhile, but eventually Karen and I were able to maneuver her back into a more comfortable position. After that, thankfully, she was quiet the rest of the night."

Today, I found Mom and Dad out of their wheelchairs, sitting in the common room side-by-side on the reclining couch holding hands, legs extended on the couch footrest. How peaceful they looked sitting so close together, staring off into space. Linda was crouched down beside Mom taking her blood pressure. "Hi Vicki, nice to see you!" (Our visits didn't often overlap.)

She offered me her weekly assessment report. "Well, I just took your Mom's blood pressure and it's 120 over 80, which is slightly higher than it was a few days ago. She weighed in below 95 pounds today."

One look at Mom confirmed she was indeed only a shadow of her former self.

"Your mom hasn't had a bowel movement in a week," continued Linda, "probably the result of her minuscule food intake. She's been drinking some fluids, but not enough to keep her from evident signs of dehydration. She's had a decreased urine output, and you can see her eyes are a little sunken, her mouth is kind of dry and tacky, and she has a general lethargy about her," as she gestured toward Mom.

Gently lifting up Mom's feet, she showed me some new bedsores, saying, "The bottom of the feet are the second most common area to develop bedsores after the buttocks. Whenever skin is pressed between a bone and hard object, such as her wheelchair footrest, these pressure sores can develop."

"Do you think they hurt her? They look painful!"

"Based on your mom's reactions, I would guess not. She doesn't even seem to notice."

"Vicki, based on what I'm seeing here, I think my earlier estimate of your mom being with us until the spring might be a bit too optimistic." I was inclined to agree.

After Linda finished her exam and left, I joined my parents on the couch, and the three of us sat with our legs resting comfortably on the footrest while Dad and I listened to Mom chatter away. Individual words were comprehensible, but her sentences made no sense.

"Well, that was a short part of the house!" She turned her head and looked at me, as if looking for a response. Not knowing what else to do, I smiled and nodded my head. She continued with her nonsensical soliloquy.

We all held hands and at one point, Mom turned towards

Dad and said in a flirty voice, "smooch, smooch, smooch," while pursing her lips. He turned toward her and gave her a kiss. She then began to talk about her "tiny, baby boy" who was sitting next to her. I wasn't sure if she meant Dad, or if she imagined that my brother, or some other unknown person was sitting next to her. She floated back and forth between seeming to know who Dad was and not having a clue. She certainly had no clue who *I* was, or at least did not give me the impression that she knew me. Despite not knowing me, however, she didn't seem to be bothered by my presence.

Maybe she finally had no more inner demons during the day, and was dwelling in a better mental place. I only heard about the evenings second-hand, and perhaps that negative behavior would eventually calm down too, as the days progressed.

There were days I felt disjointed, as if life had taken a curve into the surreal. I occasionally awakened in the morning remembering dreams from the night before, dreams of interacting with Mom and Dad as they were about 20 years ago. Momentarily confused, I promptly and dejectedly realized that it was only a dream, not the reality in which I currently lived. The dream evaporated as I was rapidly brought back to this time and place with the absoluteness that I'd never have another "real" conversation with my mother. There was no way to ask her advice, or listen to her tell me about her day. I had lost my mother in every way but physical touch, and even then, she looked at me with no recognition, and I wondered, who did she think I was? Did she even think? What would it like to be lost in her state of being? I surmised that she no longer thought in terms of me being someone she knew (her daughter) in the same sense that I might look at her and think she was my mother. She was clinging to life on another plane of existence. A mantle of despair enshrouded me.

FORTY-NINE
Tears of Love

One afternoon in mid-January, I forgot to call the facility to see if Mom was awake before I left my house. Upon arrival at Tendercare Cottages, the first thing I noticed was that Mom's door was closed. I knew what that probably meant.

Pat confirmed my suspicions. "Your mom was up all night again sitting in the middle of her mattress, talking to herself. She only fell asleep around 7 this morning."

She accompanied me as I carefully opened the door and saw Mom lying on her mattress, mostly naked. Her pajama bottoms were tangled around her calves and she had removed her pajama top altogether. The room was around 80 degrees, so at least she wasn't cold. Even though I knew she hadn't been eating much for the past six weeks, it was still a shock to see her small, naked body. She was emaciated. The bone at the bottom of her rib cage protruded like it was on the verge of poking through the skin, her ribs beneath clearly evident. Her shoulders looked like jagged mountain peaks and her hipbones formed miniature knobby rolling hills, skin over bone. The skin of her diminutive arms hung slack. There was very little, if any, fat left on her body. I had read about and seen pictures of skeleton-like people, but this was the first time I had witnessed it in person. Her body was following her mind; she was disappearing, and that reality put a lump in my throat. I wanted to rush over to where she lay, hug her, and let her know that I loved her, but thought if I did, her fragile bones might crumble.

Pat and I sat down beside her, one of us on each side, and she called Mom's name, "Trudy?"

Mom's eyes were open, so I leaned over her and said, "Hi Mom," and she actually answered with a mumbled, "Hi, sweetie." How unexpected. It had been weeks since I felt she had known me, and now she seemed to realize I was sitting beside her. I smiled inside and out, thankful for this gift. I leaned down and kissed her cheek and she made kissing sounds with her puckered lips into the air back towards me.

After a time, the caregiver left us, and as I sat beside her and stroked first her cheek and then her hair; my tears began to fall freely at the sight of this ethereal being. I held her hand, leaned over, and kissed her again. She pulled my hand to her lips and kissed it, and then kissed it a second time. The years of friction, anger, and frustration in our relationship suddenly dissolved. Past hurts no longer held any meaning. What was left was pure and palpable love. I told her over and over that I loved her, and as I held her hand, and realized, yet again, how grateful I was to be with her as she embarked on her final journey from this world to whatever lay beyond. "Mom, it's okay for you to leave us anytime, whenever you are ready. We'll be all right." I don't know if she really heard me or understood what I meant, but she went peacefully back to sleep and I continued my vigil beside her. I meditated on our relationship over the years, and how it was often stormy. Despite the friction that we often felt, I was very aware of how much she loved, protected, and took care of me as a child. Sitting next to her, I repeatedly spoke the words, "Mom, you are the best mother ever. I am so thankful that you are in my life."

Again, I'll never know if she could hear me, but somehow, I believe she could; even if she couldn't process the words, I believe she absorbed my sentiment through some form of energetic osmosis, my words blanketing her in love.

As I sat there, thoughts of my quickly approaching trip to Egypt, along with my anxiety at traveling so far, weighed ponderously on my mind. It was nearly impossible for me to even think about leaving town, let alone the country. I wondered how long Mom could continue like this, but of course, I had no idea, and ultimately, no control.

I felt very alone as the only family member experiencing this passage with Mom. It was a solitary feeling, and I wished in that moment I had someone else with whom to share it. I think how helpful it must be to have an involved sibling or family member to help shoulder the burden of this painful journey. In spite of my husband's loving support, I still struggled with a profound loneliness because my brother disengaged entirely from the process of my parents' decline, leaving the role of "supportive sibling" vacant. I was left with the next best alternative: I wrote. I wrote to let go of the pain, I wrote to feel less crazy, and I ultimately wrote to try to make sense of it all.

With my emotions nearly exhausted, I left Mom's room, suddenly realizing I hadn't spent any time with my father. I went off in search of him, and found him nonchalantly wheeling himself down the long corridor that runs the length of the facility. I steered him back towards the common living area and sat down on the couch, positioning his wheelchair next to me. He looked up at me and asked, "How old is Ray?"

Thinking quickly, I responded, "Do you mean your cousin, Ray?"

"Yes."

"Hmm, I don't really know, but I think he's older than you. What was his last name (*as I have forgotten*)?"

"Jensen," he responded right away.

Once he said the name, it immediately resonated with me that he was absolutely right. Sometimes my dad surprised me with his ability to conjure up long-term memories. Short-term memory was another matter, however; he still wanted to get up and walk and talked about that daily, even though he hadn't walked in over three years. He continued to re-sourcefully find ways to escape his wheelchair.

Because of his easy-going nature, Dad continued to be a favorite of the caregivers, and they enjoyed telling me sto-ries about his exploits. One day, he convinced someone to give him a pencil, which enabled him to unlock his seat belt. Luckily, he was being watched and did not get far once he had the seat belt unfastened. A different day, they found him proudly sitting on the toilet, pants around his ankles, still at-tached to the wheelchair and seat belt. Since I didn't witness this sight first-hand, I can only imagine him with the seat belt still around his neck, attached to the wheelchair dangling be-side him at a cockeyed angle. It remained a mystery how he managed to end up in that position without falling. Because of his continued attempts to pull the seat belt over his head, the caregivers began tying the end of it to the side of his chair. That seemed to work.

On a very cold January evening, Jody and Karen noticed that a resident's bedroom door leading outside was standing open, and when they went to investigate, saw my father out-side with no shoes or coat, wheeling himself aimlessly about in his chair. When the caregivers went outside to retrieve him, he told them he was "really cold."

Unlike Mom, I was told Dad continued to have a good appetite, and food was usually something he asked me about when I was there. "When is breakfast ... when is dinner?" then again, "When is breakfast?" He was always ready to eat.

FIFTY
Outburst

Because of our impending departure to Egypt, I started
visiting Mom and Dad even more often. Yesterday, I decided
to bring a few more of my mother's possessions home with
me. Mechanically, I loaded the items into the trunk of my
car. When I arrived home, I opened the back door, and saw
Lionel was already home from work. My first words were,
"Could you please help me unload some stuff of Mom's from
the trunk?"

He, of course, graciously did just that. In some ways, I
was numb and out of touch with how emotionally fragile I
was feeling. So was he when he sarcastically, yet playfully,
looked at me and said, "And, hello to you too," implying that
I hadn't really greeted him. In an instant the spigot came on
full force and tears flowed abundantly down my cheeks. He
quickly realized his faux pas and apologized, but it was too
late—it took me nearly 15 minutes to pull myself back together. My mental state seemed to teeter precariously on an
emotional cliff these days, with tears only a blink away. Most
days I successfully distanced myself and could maintain a
facade, but not this particular day.

Over lunch today, I described my mother's recently developed heel sores, commenting, "What is most interesting is
that the sores are on her heels, and her heels don't even touch
the ground."

"Her heels don't touch the ground?"

I wasn't sure if he was teasing me or just dense, so I stuck
my slippered foot up on the edge of the kitchen table to illus-
trate that I meant the heel on the bottom of her foot.

He said, "Pee—u, putting your feet on the table."

I exploded, "This is NOT funny. I am serious. How can you joke about this?!" I spoke more sharply than I intended. My patience was obviously in short-supply.

Lionel was visibly taken aback by my second emotional outburst in only two days. Was my sanity slipping? What force was at work causing me to react in such a manner over something so trivial? Unfortunately for Lionel, he was bearing the brunt of my overly histrionic state.

In order to calm myself, I found comfort sitting on the floor in a corner downstairs in our home, wrapped in a quilt, crying like a small child upset by a broken favorite toy. When we talked later, I described my feelings of not being taken seriously. I simply could not joke about this particular situation. For me, it was part of discussing her imminent death, but he perceived the conversation much differently and thought we were continuing with our bantering discussion of other topics during lunch. I had switched gears and left him behind. He was apologetic and asked me to say something like, "What I want to talk about now is serious for me," before I launched into anything to do with that topic again, as a reminder to him not to joke or take lightly any conversation regarding my mother. I also was apologetic for my unexpected outburst, recognizing I was on some sort of melodramatic rollercoaster.

Embarrassed by losing my cool in a manner of seconds, I wondered if I had become maladjusted. Was this behavior out of the ordinary? Should I be concerned about my *own* mental health? Why was I acting this way and lashing out toward my main support person? I hoped this would be a phase that passed quickly

Lessons Learned

Let your spouse or support person/people know when you are feeling emotionally drained, so that you can try to avoid emotional outbursts. More importantly, don't try to stuff down all your emotions during this painful journey; it will be better for your mental health if you have a healthy outlet, whether it be talking with family or friends, exercising or meditation, or just simply taking some extra relaxation time for yourself.

FIFTY-ONE
Lost Identity

"Hi Pat, how are things today?"

"Hi Vicki. Well, your mom never even got up yesterday and then slept all night! No one can remember the last time she slept all night. She actually got up this morning, drank two tall glasses of water, and ate half of a pancake!"

"Really? That's great."

"You should have seen her an hour ago. We found her lying on her back on her mattress with one leg pointing to the ceiling in what I would call some sort of ballet pose," she chuckled. "My thought was, well, at least she's pretty flexible. Hey, maybe we can get her a job with the Rockettes!" she joked.

"Hah! I'm on my way out there for a visit. See you in a bit," I said.

"Okay, sounds good. Your mom is relaxing on the couch with your dad at the moment."

Fifteen minutes later, I walked through the door at Tendercare Cottages, and spied my parents still resting quietly on the couch, feet up on the footrest, covered by a blanket. They were both sound asleep. Even if they weren't aware of each other on a conscious level, I was nearly positive I sensed some sort of connection, a comfort and a familiarity that existed between them as they sat there together. I was reminded again what a blessing it was for them to have each other, at least on some level. I attempted to wake them, and Dad opened his eyes long enough to say "hello," but Mom was in a deep sleep and unresponsive. It made for a rather short visit.

I returned the next day for a visit, hoping to find them awake for a change. Pat waved at me from the kitchen and relayed, "The Hospice nurse was here earlier. She says your mom weighs 91 pounds today." That came as no surprise, knowing she was barely eating. Mom had become incontinent and constipated at the same time, the constipation a direct result of her lack of calories. She was again receiving a stool softener to help things along.

At that moment, Dad woke up and called, "Oh! I have to go potty!" Pat walked over, transferred him into his wheelchair, and off they went to his bathroom.

I sat down beside Mom, leaned over and kissed her and said "Hi Mom," to which she replied, "Fried chicken!" She giggled, and I kissed her cheek some more.

She mumbled something about "getting ready for school."

I asked her, "Is your dad there?"

"No, I haven't seen him for awhile."

"Is you mom there?"

"Of course she is here."

"Remember how tasty your mom's chicken gravy made with fresh milk tastes, ladled over a mound of mashed potatoes? Along with her crispy fried chicken? Just thinking about it makes my mouth water!"

She looked at me and said, "I can't eat too much because I don't want to get fat."

"You don't have to worry about that! There is absolutely no chance of that happening."

Changing the subject, she asked, "What is my name?"

"Trudy!"

Mom giggled.

"What's so funny?"

"I'm just so happy that's my name."

She didn't retain it, of course, because later I asked her who she was and she didn't know. I told her again, and she attempted to repeat her name several times, but she couldn't seem to make her tongue work in order to put the sounds together to form her name. It was good to see her content though, even if she had apparently lost her identity.

I smothered her with kisses, and told her how much I loved her many, many times today. At one point, she asked, "Where is my sweet girl?"

"Here I am!" I said as I snuggled in closer to her.

Pat walked by where we were sitting and asked, "Honey, are you hungry?"

Mom exclaimed, "Yes! Can I have ice cream?" Pat made a beeline to the freezer to retrieve some.

As the caregiver began feeding her, Mom worried, "Oh, I'm afraid I'm going to spoil my dinner. What are we having for dinner?"

Her eyes got as big as saucers when Pat said, "Chicken casserole," and when I added, "with blueberry muffins and Jell-O," her eyes got even bigger and rounder.

"I shouldn't eat any more ice cream then. I'll wait for dinner."

Pat just rolled her eyes and said, "Yeah, she says that now, but when we set the plate in front of her, she just looks at it." I did have a hint of success managing to help her drink some grape juice and water, however.

Our trip to Egypt was four days away. Pat told me Mom was awake until 5 a.m., so when I arrived around 3 p.m. today, she was just waking up. She had a short-sleeved shirt on, and her skinny, wrinkly arms were striking. My energetic dad, meanwhile, was maneuvering his wheelchair around in circles, getting his daily "exercise." Without thinking, I broke one of the Alzheimer's "rules" and I pointed to Dad and asked Mom who he was, and she looked at him and after a moment of reflection, said, "Mr. Merry-berry." She was in a pretty talkative mood, at least for a few minutes, before she suddenly fell sound asleep while sitting in her wheelchair.

"Hey, Dad, how's life treating you today?" I was watching him as he wheeled around the dining area.

His reply was a toothy grin. A man of few words, my father, but he got the point across just fine.

FIFTY-TWO
Last Goodbye?

On January 30, the day before our scheduled departure to Egypt, I made one last visit to say goodbye to Mom and Dad, all the while mentally torturing myself with the thought that it might be my last goodbye to either of them.

It was difficult, and I spent most of my time saying goodbye in my mind, memorizing what it felt like to hold their shriveled hands in mine, kiss their wrinkled faces, and hug my mother's tiny, frail body. I trudged out of the facility in a slight daze, not conscious of putting one foot in front of the other.

Would I see them both again? Was I making a poor life choice? Would I successfully cope with the self-imposed guilt?

FIFTY-THREE
Pharaonic Tales

"Once you start to cross the street, do not back up!" my daughter Jill instructed as we made our way across five or possibly seven (it was difficult to tell) chaotic lanes of traffic on a congested Cairo city street. "People assume you're moving forward and drive accordingly. Once you've vacated the space, a car will quickly fill it!" *Just like life, we could only go forward. There was no backing up.* Sighing, I wondered how my parents were getting along at Tendercare Cottages. They also could only move forward to the inevitable end that awaits us all. I hoped they were okay. The staff had my e-mail address and so far, there had been no e-mail from Tendercare Cottages. I hoped that was a good sign. I forced myself to shake off thoughts of home and returned to the present, surrounded by Lionel, our children, and their significant others, attempting to stay focused on the here and now. Being together was the high point of our trip.

Here we were in a city of more than 20 million people, crowded together in a megalopolis that seemed ready to implode at any moment. The crumbling facades of colonial architecture provided a glimpse into the genteel Cairo of another time. Today, traffic, combined with the mass of humanity, assailed the senses at every turn; this was not a city for the faint of heart. Poverty stared back at us from every angle, hardship written into the deep creases on the faces of street-side vendors, an acridly sweet aroma emanating from their pushcarts filled with roasting nuts. And the noise! There was a continuous stream of honking cars passing by in every direction, both day and night.

En route to our next tour destination, we became even more acutely aware of the gap between rich and poor. We watched a crush of people queuing for free government-issued bread, beggars crowding the sidewalks, and children joyfully playing soccer in the narrow alleyways, all witnessed from the comfort of our air-conditioned, chauffeured tour company van. In spite of the evident poverty, Egyptians we encountered along the way were both welcoming and kind, and proud that we were visiting their country. I chuckled as I imagined Mom's "tsk, tsk, tsk-ing" at the lack of pristine public restrooms, as well as the dirty, littered, and crowded streets, asking me, "Why would you possibly want to go to Egypt? And besides that, why in the *world* would Jill want to *live* there?" It seemed my thoughts returned to my parents no matter where I was or what I was doing.

We visited the pyramids at Dahshur, Sakkara, and Giza. Surprisingly, the Giza pyramids, the most well known, are fairly close to downtown Cairo. Even from a distance, they are mammoth in size, rising triumphantly above the Cairo skyline. These were not the first pyramids on our tour that morning, however. On our way to Sakkara, the first site we visited, we traveled along a surprisingly desolate desert road, passing through numerous small villages along the narrow Nile canals. Greenery followed along the canals, but shortly beyond was golden sand of the Sahara Desert, as far as the eye could see.

The road then took us through the open desert for a short distance until we arrived at the base of the famed Steppe Pyramid at Sakkara. Later that morning we traveled to the Giza Plateau, anxiously anticipating our visit to the grand edifice of the Cheops Pyramid, also commonly referred to as the Great Pyramid. The largest of the three pyramids comprising the Giza Necropolis, it's the oldest of the seven wonders of the ancient world, and the only one that remains largely intact. As we stepped out of our tour van, a silence washed over all of us as we stood staring, dumbfounded by the pyramids' sheer size, and completely in awe of the ancient culture that constructed them.

It was astonishing to me that no one knows for certain how or why the pyramids were built. One thing was certain—the pyramids, a testament to man's ability to reach across time and space, have long outlasted the humans who engineered them. I paused a moment to reflect on how many of us have gone before, and how many are yet to come, reminded that although we turn to dust, our achievements often live on.

What would be my parents' legacy? I reflected, as we walked near these vast, venerable structures. My mind filled with thoughts of old furniture, pictures and a trinket or two. In the end, I guess, that's all most of us leave behind. On that depressing note, I suddenly had an inspiration … *Wait! They are leaving us behind! Their family is their legacy! We, who carry their memories and love in our hearts forever.*

We traveled by boat up the Nile to Luxor. We were up quite early most mornings to see the historic sites and avoid the afternoon heat. One day, we awakened at 4:30 a.m. to visit the Valley of the Kings, where many tombs of ancient pharaohs have been uncovered over the past century. It was already stiflingly hot at 8:30 a.m. as we arrived in this hilly, dry desert region. We were allowed to walk around part of the area and visit some of the tombs on our own. Walking down into these tombs, we were quickly enveloped first by the welcome cool air, and secondly by how heavy and stale it felt. We were amazed by the intricate artwork on the walls, each tomb decorated in a different artistic style. We soon realized construction of these tombs probably began the moment a new pharaoh came into power, in order to have enough time to finish them before the pharaoh passed on. How different life was 2,500 years ago.

Ancient Egyptians believed that when we die, we merely cross over to another existence, and for our new life we must take belongings from this world. The pharaohs, seen as gods, were believed to die and be reborn every day with the rising and setting of the sun. For people important enough to be mummified and buried in a tomb, all needs for their future were met by filling the tomb with their chariot, furniture, jewelry, pottery, food, and even mummified animals, such as cats and horses. It was obvious they felt very strongly about an afterlife, and unlike our culture, thought they could take their wealth and possessions with them. I pondered what Mom and Dad might think about this idea.

I found myself gazing at the mummified remains of King Tut, speculating once again, what if Mom died while I was gone? I reassured myself with the morbid thought that Hospice had told me they could keep her body in storage for up to two weeks. If the ancient Egyptians could preserve a body for thousands of years, I guess I could relax and believe that our modern culture would be able to keep Mom's body waiting for a couple of weeks.

FIFTY-FOUR
The Stuffed Animal "Napper"

We safely returned from our trip to Egypt, and to my great relief, Mom and Dad appeared much the same as when I had last visited. In spite of how much I had seen and done in the past two weeks, for them, time seemed to have stood still. The first thing I learned from Pat was that this morning Mom had eaten some scrambled eggs, and at the noon meal drunk some water. Another of life's small victories! I walked over to where she was sitting in her wheelchair with her feet up on the couch and gave her a hug and kiss.

Dad was sitting in his wheelchair in his room, pushed right up against his bed staring longingly at it, as he often did, probably wishing he were in it. After greeting Mom, I went into his room, gave him a similar hug and kiss hello, and he immediately asked me, "Could you help me into my bed?" I explained, "It isn't time quite yet, Dad, so how about if you join Mom and me in the living room?"

I wheeled him out next to where Mom was sitting, and he sat there looking at her with a most intense expression on his face. Mom looked over at me and said, "See how mean he looks?" I must admit, he did look rather fierce.

He asked me, "Would you yank on this and pull it off?" referring to his seat belt.

"I'm sorry Dad, but I can't do that; you see, I don't have the special key to unlock it." (I was forever trying to come up with "good" reasons for why I wouldn't help him unlock his seat belt). A bit disgruntled, he nodded his head in tacit defeat. How frustrated he must have felt! Before I knew it, he had wheeled himself around back into his room, positioning himself in much the same position facing his bed where I had found him only minutes before. Evidently he was much happier sitting in his room staring at his bed than socializing with Mom and me, so I let him be.

Pat told me that Dad had now resorted to asking for forks to try and get his seat belt off, so they had to be extra careful he didn't wheel away with his fork at mealtime. It seemed his primary goal these days was to "escape," either from his seat belt or out any door of any room to which he gained access. He certainly enjoyed roaming around, the same as he did at Cedar Grove, and hanging out in other people's rooms, often to their chagrin.

While cleaning up in the kitchen a few days ago, Pat told me she heard Martha, one of the residents, shouting, "Help! There's a man in my room undressing!" and looked up to find Martha chasing Dad out of her room, waving her cane behind him. Luckily, Pat was right there to rescue him from Martha's wrath.

The caregiver went on to share, "Your Dad and I were playing the Crazy Eights card game a couple of days ago, and I'm a witness here to tell you that he won more than one game! He's much sharper than we suspected. You know, we didn't even think he could talk when he moved here!" Since Dad didn't talk much, it gave the impression he might not be "with it," when he probably was much more aware than any of us gave him credit for.

Shelly happened to be there today, and walked over to where I was talking with Pat. She joined our conversation, remarking, "Interestingly enough, lately your dad's been a lot more alert and active both day and night. He isn't sleeping well, though, and we aren't sure what's caused the change. He spent most of the last six months here sleeping, and now he's almost like a whole different person with all this energy!" I agreed with her. When I visited, he did seem to be spending a lot less time with his chin resting on his chest and with eyes closed.

"While it's good to see him more interactive, it's causing some issues during the night because he wakes up and tries to crawl out of bed and then falls. So far, we've been lucky he hasn't injured himself, but it's a concern. He acts restless, so I thought maybe pain is waking him, but he denies having any pain. I did a physical exam, and his heart sounds fine, his blood pressure falls within the normal range, and his oxygen saturation readings are better than mine! We'll continue to monitor and keep a close eye on him for any signs of pain and to leave his door open slightly at night so we can hear him if he starts to stir. I've suggested that the caregivers just go ahead and get him up, put him in his wheelchair and bring him out into the kitchen for a snack with the hope that he'll go back to bed after that." I nodded agreement with this plan. *How familiar –his night behavior was beginning to sound a lot like Mom's.*

Pat then shared another story. "Yeah, well, the other evening, Jody, who was working the night shift, put him in his wheelchair when he woke up and brought him into the kitchen with her. She had to leave him for a few moments to help Karen attend to another resident, and when they came back into the kitchen, he was nowhere to be found."

"You're kidding! Where was he? Had he gone outside again?" No one had told me about this.

"Well, Jody and Karen did a room-by-room search, and when they finally found him, he'd collected what they called a 'herd of stuffed animals' from the other residents' rooms. They said he acted *very* pleased with himself. Once they could stop laughing, I guess they had quite a time figuring out where each of the stuffed animals lived."

When I later asked Dad about collecting all the stuffed animals. He said, "Yeah, I had a whole wagon load!" and smiled at me, obviously pleased by his escapade.

As my thoughts returned to the present moment, I turned my attention back to Mom, tuning in to her babble. At one point, she looked at me and said clearly, "You look a lot like Vicki."

"Well, Mom, that's because I am Vicki." This was an example of a fleeting, yet unpredictable, lapse into recognition. Some of her sentences, like that one, were understandable, but many were interspersed with gibberish that made understanding her difficult, if not impossible.

She did like conversing and asking questions, which was always challenging when I couldn't understand the question. I tried to take her cue as to whether I should nod in agreement or not.

Driving home after the visit, I acknowledged to myself that there was no sign from either of them that they'd even noticed I hadn't visited for two weeks. I had to admit, this assuaged my guilt, to some degree.

Lesson Learned

Try to maintain a light heart. Some comic relief can be a welcome reprieve from the stress of this journey!

FIFTY-FIVE
Stains and Two Pounds of Sugar

Today I found myself yearning to call Mom, ask her advice, and update her on my life, and then grieving because I couldn't. This realization evoked such a profound sense of loss. No longer could I hope to rely on my mother's wisdom; instead, I have now moved to the front of the line, and it's my children calling to ask me how to remove that pesky stain from their shirts.

This afternoon I attended the graveside service and reception for an 87-year-old friend of my parents who was also the parent of my friend Jackie. Her father, Ray, had passed away at home, sitting in his favorite chair. He was beginning to need more and more care, but before it became necessary to move him to a skilled-nursing center, he made his own exit, quietly and peacefully. In light of the emotionally difficult experience I was having with my own parents, I couldn't help but think, *how fortunate for them all*!

Julie, a mutual friend of both Jackie and me, also attended the service. Her parents died together when their small airplane crashed almost 30 years ago, when she was still in her twenties. While we were at the service Julie turned to me and said, "Sometimes I think about losing my parents when I did, and then look at what you and Jackie have gone through with your parents, not to mention what *they* have endured. I wonder what my parents might have chosen had they had a choice. Would they have wanted to bear what your parents are going through? From my perspective, I think being able to have my parents with me longer, even though it can be very difficult at the end, is still better than the shock of having lost them both so young. They were only 49 and 51 years old when they died."

That certainly put things into perspective, especially when I considered the fact that I was already older than Julie's parents when they died. After the funeral reception, I stopped to visit Mom and Dad. Dad was scooting about the facility in his wheelchair. He thoroughly enjoyed my greeting of kisses, hugs, and handholding. After dusting some food particles off his shirt, I moved on to find Mom sleeping on the couch, looking more shrunken than last week. Cell by cell, she was unmistakably disappearing. The wrinkles in her face were becoming more pronounced as her skin sagged from the lack of subcutaneous fat. For several moments, I became absorbed with stroking her silky, almost diaphanous ear lobes. I had never witnessed such paper-thin lobes. Something required me to physically touch what my eyes were observing, as if I had to caress them in order to make them real. Her skin reminded me of delicate porcelain, almost translucent in its appearance.

Pat told me Mom had only a bit of water to drink so far today. She was sleeping more and more. Each day that I'd called this week to see if it was a good time to visit, the caregivers told me she was sleeping. Today I went anyway. I awakened her and she babbled something about "the kids eating their lunch up on the hill." I didn't know if she was remembering attending her country school or what was in her mind. She talked about not getting her "two pounds of sugar" because she didn't bring her "card." I was wondering if she was thinking of ration cards during World War II. It was difficult to say, because most of her sentences started out semi-coherent, but then trailed off into gibberish mid-sentence.

Mom drifted in and out of sleep throughout my visit. Dad continued meandering around the common area in his wheelchair, stopping to say "Hi" on every round, with side trips back to his room to look longingly at his bed. He acted bored and restless today, like he was looking for something to do. When I left, he was digging around in his nightstand drawer, which contained a thin book, a shoehorn and a note-pad. I asked for a hug, and he was very agreeable to that, and a kiss or two. I felt so sad for him today, realizing that his life had been reduced to rummaging through a drawer and wheeling his wheelchair around in circles. Mom continued to sleep peacefully on the couch as I left the facility to return home. There were times like this that I wanted to scream in frustration or throw plates against the wall. *Why* were the last years of life like this for my parents?

FIFTY-SIX
The Power of Touch

While visiting my parents today, I was awed by the infinite power of human touch. Tendercare Cottages called me late this afternoon. "Even though she hasn't eaten or taken in any liquid in a couple of days, your Mom is awake and pretty talkative, if you want to come over." I promptly left my house to drive to the facility.

When I arrived, Mom was curled up asleep on the couch. *Shoot! I had hoped she would still be awake when I got here.* As per usual, Dad was wheeling aimlessly about the facility in his wheelchair. I sat down with Mom on the couch and snuggled right down close to her, and attempted to talk with her. Pat came over and helped me wake her up. Mom talked about being "a bad girl" and "leaving." Nothing she uttered made much sense, so I simply sat and held her hand and watched her sleep. Dad wheeled by the back of the couch and laid his hand on top, so with my other free hand, I grabbed his hand. He smiled and gave it a squeeze. Here I was linked to both my parents, hands within hands. This profound feeling of connection suddenly gave way to the insight that one of these days, holding the hands of both my living parents will be at an end. Tears lurked at the corners of my eyes as I tried my best not to fixate on that thought.

We sat like that for a time, until Mom blurted out, "I'm thirsty." Like saying "bomb" in an airport, that was one statement that was sure to get immediate attention and action. Pat hurriedly brought over a glass of water, and I attempted to help Mom take a sip. She said, "Bleck, tastes bad. No more." I encouraged her to give it another try. Her next comment was, "No, not cold enough," and she refused to take any more. The caregiver told me she'd encourage her to drink something later at supper.

Mom's face had lost more shape this week, and just when I imagined she couldn't look any thinner or show more sagging and wrinkles as she disappeared, she did. Mom was growing more diminutive and fragile with each passing day. Today, she *did* hold my hand tightly, however, so evidently not all her strength was gone. I held close the belief she knew it was me who was snuggling next to her this afternoon.

FIFTY-SEVEN
Get Me a Screwdriver!

On Leap Year Day, February 29, I stopped at Tendercare Cottages without calling first. It had been three days since I last visited. I had begun to feel a sense of urgency about visiting often. When I walked in, there sat Mom in a corner of the common area in her wheelchair, head on her chest, asleep, or at least giving the appearance of sleep. Dad was nowhere to be seen. I walked over to Mom, knelt down, kissed her and said "hello." No response. I attempted to get her to open her eyes. Bleary looking and red-rimmed, her eyes opened halfway to peer outward with a rather glazed-over, vacant look. Her face was ashen-colored. *Oh!* I nearly gasped aloud as my intuition shrieked the end was exceedingly close. I released an audible sigh as I offered her my hand, which she grasped in hers, and quietly said "Ooh," because it was cold. Finally, here was a sound of life in a fairly lifeless-looking body. She was so slight my fingers could nearly encircle her entire upper arm. Her bony shoulders were even taller mountain peaks than before. Her head appeared too large for her body, and *it* wasn't very big. She mumbled softly to me, speaking unintelligible words. I kissed and caressed her, and repeatedly told her, "I love you mama. Your girl is here to see you." There seemed to be little awareness on her part. I wasn't sure if she was asleep or awake, or in some semi-conscious state between the two.

Pat came over to us, and I took the opportunity to ask her, "Do you know where my dad is?" Adding a bit of levity to my day, she said, "Oh, probably in some lady's room. He's been in and out of all the women's rooms today. Earlier we were talking about wine, women, and song, and asked your dad which he would choose, and he said, 'a little of all three!'" Sure enough, a minute later the caregiver was wheeling him out of another woman's room and over to where Mom and I were. Nodding in Mom's direction, I asked him, "Do you know who I'm talking to?" He shook his head no. Pat informed me that he had been holding one of the other resident's hands earlier in the afternoon. He seemed to have more or less forgotten who Mom was. Because of his dementia, I couldn't possibly be irritated with him, and I suspected he would have no trouble adjusting to her being gone, someday soon. Maybe that was a blessing in disguise.

He quickly got bored with us and wheeled off to another part of the room. Mom seemed to want to sleep, so I walked the few steps over to where Dad was temporarily located. He smiled sweetly at me and asked for a screwdriver.

"What do you want a screwdriver for?" I asked, knowing exactly what he wanted it for.

"To take this thing off!" (Referring to his seat belt, just as I expected.)

"Well, then what would you do?"

"I would take it off."

"And then?"

"I would get up and go."

"Where would you go?"

"Uh, I don't know."

"Well, you need a plan as to where you'd go. Where would you like to go?"

"Hmm, I hadn't thought about that."

"Do you remember that you can't walk?"

"Yes."

"The reason you have the seat belt is to protect you from falling and hurting yourself."

"Oh."

And so it went as the conversation repeated itself several times. As we were entering the fourth iteration of this conversation, Pat approached us.

"Get me a screwdriver!"

"Sorry, we can't give you a screwdriver," answered the caregiver. "What do you want it for?" (She also knew what he would say.)

"So I can get this thing off."

"We can't take it off. You have that on for your own good, so you don't get hurt. How about you have supper first, and then one of us will take it off and you can sit on the couch and watch *The Price is Right*?"

"You won't be able to get it off!"

"Yes, we will. Remember, we have a magic tool to remove it?"

Begrudgingly, he grunted his acceptance.

A few seconds later he blurted out, to no one in particular, "Get me a screwdriver!"

Oh, the futility of it all. I went back over to where Mom was sitting, as I could hear her mumbling again. She was very difficult to understand today. I moved my ear closer to her mouth in an attempt to glean any sort of meaning from her words. "I heard her ask for water!" I exclaimed. Pat and I immediately got a small glass, and put about an inch of water in it. Mom wanted ice, so we added ice. She took one baby sip and pushed the glass away.

"Has she eaten anything lately?" I asked Pat.

She responded, "We gave her a bowl of pears for breakfast, which she promptly picked up and dumped upside down on the table. Then she ate two tiny pieces of pear off the table. At lunch she just looked at the food. She hasn't really had much of anything to drink in the past few days, either. She's probably eaten about 5 percent of her food this week." She was talking about five percent of only tablespoons that they serve her. I was yet again amazed that a human being could continue to subsist on so little.

"Mom, God is waiting for you, whenever you are ready," I whispered to her. I received no response.

FIFTY-EIGHT
Evening Visit

Today, March 3, I was finished at work and home for lunch when the telephone rang. When I answered, I was greeted by the voice of Tendercare Cottage's nurse. I braced myself for the news I had been expecting to come at any moment.

"Hello, this is Shelly."

"Yes?" I said with dread in my voice, fearing news of my mother's imminent death.

"I'm not calling about your mother, but your father." Immense relief washed over me. It was surprising that a single instant could make me feel so grateful that I don't yet have to face the inevitable. That moment passed though, as I was filled with concern for my father.

"Oh, really? Is he okay?"

"Well, his hand is swollen, and black and blue, and no one seems to know what happened. He doesn't complain of pain until I do deep tissue pressure, so I don't think it's broken."

After some discussion, it was decided that Lionel and I would drive over to Tendercare Cottages after he arrived home from work this evening to examine Dad and see if we needed to take him to the hospital emergency department. We walked into Tendercare Cottages around 7 p.m. and found Mom sitting on the couch; she was the sole occupant of the living area. Dad was in his room in his wheelchair attempting to reach something on top of his dresser. Upon examination, Lionel determined that nothing appeared broken, but it was certainly swollen and tender. The most plausible explanation was that Dad's hand had somehow gotten caught in the wheel of his chair as he was rolling around. It had no doubt happened sometime last night, because the afternoon caregivers said he was okay when they left work yesterday. Lionel determined that a splint would immobilize and protect his hand, and hopefully help the pain Dad was now experiencing with movement. Lionel drove back to his clinic and retrieved a splint, while I remained at Tendercare Cottages with Mom and Dad.

Dad was a busybody tonight. Jody, who was working alone this evening, decided to help one of the residents take a shower as long as I was there to look after Mom and Dad, the only two residents I saw the entire time we were there. Everyone else was already in bed.

While I was awaiting Lionel's return, and with my attention focused on Mom, I noticed my dad wheeling into Mom's room. Before I realized what he was doing (one shoe on and one shoe off), he had opened her door to the backyard and proceeded to go outside into the cold winter night. I quickly retrieved him, blocked off the door, and returned to where Mom was sitting. As I continued to wait, Dad occupied himself by scooting off down the halls. After he disappeared from view, I went to check on him and found him in another resident's room attempting to open her door to the outside. He was certainly determined and resourceful. I brought him out of this room and encouraged him to come into the living area with Mom and me. He sat patiently for a minute or two before he was off in another direction, attempting to open the door into yet another resident's room. I admonished, "No, you can't go in there." He replied, matter-of-factly, "Yes, I can. I need to get a coat." I redirected him back towards *his* own room. He then attempted to go outside by opening his door to the backyard, but didn't make it very far, as we had strategically placed his recliner in front of the door. At most, it only opened a couple of inches. I suddenly had a deeper understanding of what the facility described to me as his "restless behavior." What a handful! He reminded me of my children when they were little.

Between episodes of chasing after my dad, I sat with Mom, who was quite talkative this evening. She was also a little restless and picking at the quilt covering her, and poking around inside her shirt. I thought maybe her bra strap had slipped down so I poked around inside her shirt myself, only to discover that she wasn't even wearing a bra. Oops! She was picking at imaginary items that only she could see or feel. When I touched her, she drew back, looked at me, eyes ablaze and chastised me, "You should be ashamed of yourself!" I stared back at her without comment and straightened her shirt. In a high-pitched, squeaky voice, she stared at me and said, properly self-chastised, "I'm sorry." Those were the most intelligible words she said to me all evening, except that she was thirsty. Jody brought her a small glass of water, which she drank over the course of several minutes. She then implored, "I'm so empty inside. Can I please have ice cream?" The caregiver looked at her skeptically, saying to me, "I'd be real surprised if she ate any ice cream, but I'll sure be glad to offer her some after I get your dad to bed." Jody then brought Mom her crushed up antidepressant mixed into some applesauce. Mom gagged in her attempt to swallow the concoction. She was still smacking her lips and making faces like she had a bad taste in her mouth five minutes later. As I watched her making faces and gagging noises, I wondered to myself *why* we were still forcing her take *any* pills.

By this time, Lionel had returned with the splint, which worked well to immobilize my dad's hand. We asked Dad, "Will you leave the Velcro splint on?" and he agreed he would. Knowing how much he liked removing things—from seat belts to clothing—we would see!

FIFTY-NINE
The End Draws Near

This morning, March 4, I called Linda at Hospice to ask if we could re-evaluate why we still required Mom to take *any* pills. She agreed that perhaps it wasn't necessary to continue the antidepressant, but wasn't sure about whether to discontinue the medication for Sundowner's Effect, as it might still be essential for Mom's sleep issues. She said she would check in with Mom's doctors and see what they suggested.

Linda went on to say in a tender voice, "I'm glad you phoned. You were on my list to call today. I weighed your mom this morning, and she now weighs 85 pounds (*40 pounds less than her normal weight*). I also wanted to let you know her O2 saturation levels are around 50 (*normal is 90*). My feeling is that she won't survive much longer, although everyone continues to be surprised by her stamina. When they're transferring her to the toilet or bed, she still shows an amazing amount of strength in her grip. No one knows where it's coming from, considering she really hasn't eaten anything in two weeks." *They didn't know my mother—determined to the very end!*

The Hospice nurse wanted to prepare me for what could happen at any time, possibly within the next two weeks. My intuition told me four days ago that the time was drawing near, and today's conversation confirmed it. I felt the paradox of despair and relief.

As I hung up with Linda, I knew what needed to be done next.

"Hello?" I heard my brother's familiar voice as he answered the phone. I had decided it was time to call him with an update on Mom's condition, and prepare him for what was undoubtedly coming soon.

"Hi Jack, it's Vicki." With slight hesitation, I continued, "I just wanted to call and let you know that Mom is getting closer to the end. Her O2 levels are way down, and her weight is somewhere around 85 pounds. The Hospice nurse told me it wouldn't be long, probably within the next two weeks. I wanted to give you some advance notice."

"Okay. Well, we haven't decided yet whether or not we'll come for the funeral, although I'm thinking at least I'll probably come. I'm not sure if Rhoda will though, because of the cost of plane tickets."

I couldn't believe I actually heard these words come out of his mouth. I suddenly felt quite indignant. *Not sure if he would come to the funeral? Of our own mother? How could he be unsure about something like THAT!? How could we be so different? They owned two houses, for heaven's sake; surely they could afford two plane tickets.* The years spent trying to overcome my anger and disappointment of an uninvolved sibling fell away as familiar feelings of frustration washed over me. I remained silent until I regained my composure.

We talked for a little while longer, though the rest of the conversation was a compete blur. I simply couldn't get past his statement about possibly not attending the funeral. *Was this some sort of coping mechanism he was using so he wouldn't actually have to face our mother's death?*

The unsettling interchange with my brother underscored that even though I perceived I was mentally prepared to face Mom's passing, such was not the case. That afternoon, as I relayed to Lionel the disheartening information from the Hospice nurse and the phone conversation with my brother, my voice wavered shakily and tears rolled over my cheeks. The reality of what lay ahead slammed into me full force.

SIXTY
Pucker-up

On March 5, I arrived at Tendercare Cottages to find Mom in her wheelchair in the dining area. Most of the other residents, including Dad, were off enjoying the weekly bus ride, so it was eerily quiet.

It was painful for me to look at her. I wouldn't have thought it possible, but in two days she had visibly declined even further. I ached inside as I took note of her mouth, slack and hanging open, possibly to catch more air as her ability to breathe continued to falter. Although she was slumped forward in her chair, her eyes were open, and she was softly mumbling, to no one in particular. I sensed death lurking nearby. It was in the shadows of her eyes, the sagging crevices of her skin, and the shallow breathing on her lips. I heard one coherent sentence today, and it was "I do not approve." Strange.

I held her hands, caressed her face, and ran my fingers through her hair while I softly wept. "Mom, soon you will see your mama, papa, brother, aunt, and lots of old friends. Would you like that? Please know that Dad and I will be okay, and you can go whenever you're ready." She was unresponsive today except for one moment when I said "Pucker up and give me a kiss!" And, she did! This was the only indication that she could hear me today. She was moving steadily ahead into another life, another world.

Dad returned from the bus trip with a broad smile on his face. "Hey, Dad! How was the bus ride?"

"Oh, fine, yes … fine," he replied.

"What did you see?"

"Mostly a lot of traffic," was his reply.

The facility activities director invited him to participate in the craft activity. He selected red paint, and along with two other ladies, began to paint the giant paper maché volcano the activities director had built. The plan was to put vinegar and baking soda into the caldera after they finished painting the outside, for a big show. I was not present when they added the vinegar solution, but I am told it bubbled nicely, just like a miniature volcano. It's funny how second graders and the elderly derive joy from many of the same activities. I never, ever imagined my dad participating in craft activities. He was certainly a changed man!

A friend, whose mother was in the early stages of Alzheimer's disease, stopped by Tendercare Cottages and visited with me and Mom this afternoon. Though not a family member, having her there with me to share in this experience helped my mental attitude. The three of us held hands, and we said a prayer for Mom. It was an emotional, peace-giving experience.

SIXTY-ONE
Dying Can Be a Lot of Work

It was March 6, the eve of my birthday. I awakened early with a premonition that my phone would soon ring. It didn't happen until around 9 a.m., when I was already at work, so the continual ringing only echoed throughout an empty house. Continuing to work mornings helped me cope with the waiting, and lessened the intensity of both my grief and anxiety for a few hours each day.

The strange feeling I had experienced upon awakening continued, so midway through my morning I checked my cell phone to see if I had any messages from Tendercare Cottages; I did. When I hadn't answered my phone at home, they had called my cell phone, which I hadn't heard ring. The message was simple: "When you get this message, please call us." Trepidation set in, leaving me paralyzed. I could not push the numbers on my phone. I didn't want to hear that she had died. After several minutes, the uncertainty of wondering became more unbearable than the fear of calling, so I finally made the call and learned, with relief, that Mom was still alive. She had stopped breathing momentarily, however, and "maybe" I would like to come out to the facility.

In a daze, I walked out of my office to find there was a patient waiting to see me. Trance-like, I entered the exam room and went through the motions of a somewhat surreal appointment. Afterwards, I came out of the exam room, and holding back tears, told the office staff that my mother was dying and I had to leave. They practically pushed me out the door exclaiming, "Go, go!" So, as if under a sorcerer's spell, I mechanically put on my coat, walked to my car, called my pastor/friend to meet me, and drove to Tendercare Cottages, feeling completely numb.

Mom lay curled up in the fetal position on her mattress on the floor, looking still tinier than yesterday.

I sat down beside her, gently touched and kissed her. I told her, "I love you," and she mumbled back to me, maybe she was saying she loved me as well. I couldn't understand her. I repeated, "Your mom, dad, brother, and a whole lot of your friends are waiting for you, whenever you're ready to go."

She audibly responded, "Okay."

"I'll take care of Dad and we'll be okay. Dad will join you sometime soon."

"That's wonderful!" came out very clearly, and then, "Goodbye."

She closed her eyes, and went back into her state of altered consciousness, somewhere between awake and asleep, or alive and dead. I detected an odor about her, a noxious smell that I'd never before encountered. It permeated her body—especially her breath. Was that the "smell of death" I had often read about? I always thought that "smell" was a literary embellishment. It was real.

My pastor friend arrived shortly thereafter, and joined Mom and me in her room. The two of us visited for a few minutes about my mother and her life before he asked her if it was all right if he said some prayers. She actually groaned out an "uh huh," before he read a passage from Psalm 139, and offered prayers. Our voices united in the Lord's Prayer, and the pastor administered what I surmised were the "last rites." The prayer was comforting and brought me a calming sense of peace.

As the pastor was leaving, my dear friend, Diane, arrived to offer a hug and comfort. Next, Lionel arrived, and the two of us sat silently beside Mom. Lionel stayed with me for his entire lunch break, but had to return to the office. He told me to call him if anything changed.

As the afternoon became evening, her hands took on more of a bluish hue, and her face had turned an unearthly grey. Her feet looked red and sore. She varied between chatty, sleepy, restless, and moaning. I prayed for her, sung variations of *Amazing Grace*, and *Swing Low, Sweet Chariot*. I caressed and kissed her, helped her eat ice chips, watched helplessly as she gagged with dry heaves, and kept vigil beside her as she slept. Thankfully, the caregivers gave her a suppository to stop the dry heaves, and for that I was especially grateful. She sat up several times and picked at her covers, throwing them off and talked about strange things. She very clearly counted something out loud, and then looked at the wall speaking to someone I couldn't see.

"I need to get my work done, but I'm so tired."

"Mom, it's okay, I'll do your work. You can lay down and rest now."

"Oh, can I?" I helped her lay back down on her bed.

A few minutes later, she sat up again and opened her eyes very wide. I looked at her, and said, "I love you."

She looked back at me and said unmistakably, "And I love you too." And then she lay back down.

My daughter called from her home in Egypt and asked, "Do you think Grandma would understand who I am if I talked to her?"

I said, "Yes, I really think she will. Let's try it!"

I placed the phone next to Mom's ear.

I heard Jill say, "Grandma, it's me, Jill. I'll be home in a few days, and I'll come right out to see you. I love you!"

315

Her voice was shaky and filled with tears, but I know her Grandma heard her, because she softly, but audibly mumbled in reply, "Okay, I love you too."

It was a blessing that Mom was alert enough in that moment to speak to her granddaughter. I was afraid, though, that Jill would be too late to see her Grandma alive.

By late evening I had watched Mom's corpus alternate between lying quite still with hands folded upon her chest, to mumbling and restlessly moving about. I watched patiently as she struggled with that final sleep. She had chosen to not go quietly, but continued to battle death, even though it seemed there should be no strength left in her frail and wizened body. All of Mom's caregivers continued to express complete amazement at her tenacity to hang on to life.

She slowly became more agitated as the evening wore on. I watched as she sat up and scooted around on the mattress, throwing off her covers. Speaking to no one in particular (as far as I know), I heard "I can't do this anymore," before she curled into a little ball at the foot of her mattress, motionless.

Today I learned dying could be a lot of hard work.

SIXTY-TWO
Last Goodbyes

On my birthday, March 7, I awakened early and called the facility to see how the night had gone. As I sensed she would, Mom pulled through the night okay. She's not finished with this life. I hoped it wasn't too much to ask for her not to die today. I couldn't face the thought of my mother dying on my birthday.

That afternoon she scooted around on her bed, somewhat agitated. Each time we moved her back onto her pillow in the center of the bed, within minutes she had turned sideways and crawled back over to the edge of the bed so her arms and legs hung over the side of the mattress. Her fingers and hands appeared purple now, certainly made worse by dangling them over the side of the mattress.

Very plainly she said to me, "I'm so dry, I want some water." I immediately retrieved some water and helped her sit up. I gave her the glass to hold, which was difficult for her to maneuver, but easier than me pouring the water in her mouth and choking her. She took a big sip, and within seconds began gagging, crying, and bending over in pain. I then felt completely responsible for causing her pain. The dry heaves started again, so I grabbed a towel for her to spit into, and calmed her as best I could until it passed. Pat came in and again gave her a suppository to stop the dry heaves. While she was in the room with us, she relayed a story to me. "Jody told me yesterday before she left for the weekend that your mom told her she wouldn't be seeing her again because she was going to be with her parents." This poignant comment told me that Mom still had some sort of clarity—an awareness of what was happening, and an intuition about what was to come.

My brother and sister-in-law called to tell me "Happy Birthday." That seemed a contradiction in some way, as I am not sure "happy" birthday applied. Because Mom talked to Jill yesterday, it occurred to me to offer them that same opportunity, to say their goodbyes. At first, they both seemed a little reluctant, and asked, "Do you think she'll have awareness of who we are?"

"I think she will." *Wasn't it at least worth trying? It would probably be their last chance to talk to her.*

They decided to talk to her.

My sister-in-law Rhoda was sobbing as she told Mom, "I'm so thankful that you had a son." My brother also sounded choked up as they both told her, "We love you very much." She softly murmured something unintelligible to them in reply.

Thus began a series of heart-wrenching conversations, as one by one, all my children and both of my brother's children called to wish me "Happy Birthday" and were given the opportunity to tell their grandma goodbye.

Both of my brother's daughters, Katie and Deanna, were tearful as they thanked their grandma for being the best grandmother ever, and said their goodbyes. Each of them got to hear at least a couple intelligible words, with one of my nieces hearing her say, "I've had a good, long life. I love you, too." Most of her words were soft mumbles, and we could only guess what she was trying to say. I was positive it included the words, "I love you, too" for each of them.

Before the afternoon was over, Mom had "spoken" to all five of her grandchildren, as well as her son and his wife. My younger niece, Katie, was the last to speak with her on the phone. Katie told me, "I am so sorry this is happening on your birthday. How awful it must be for you." In that moment it occurred to me that it really wasn't an "awful" birthday. It was precisely *because* of my birthday that my family received an opportunity to say goodbye, which may not have otherwise occurred. What a blessing that it was my birthday. *My* true birthday gift was the opportunity to be a witness to these heartfelt conversations of gratefulness and goodbyes to a loving and spirited mother/grandmother. Tears of love and joy cascaded freely down my cheeks as I held my cell phone to my mother's ear for these loving conversations. This particular birthday would be unforgettable.

I had the privilege of spending all these hours with Mom to love and comfort her along her final journey, "walking" alongside her with the opportunity to tell her over and over all the words I cared to say. I wouldn't be choked up with regrets of moments lost, as I was a witness to the entire journey. I held her hand, stroked her cheek, rubbed her back, and kissed her as she moved ever closer to the proverbial finish line. It was a tangible good-bye. I knew this time with her was easing the grieving process, and giving me closure far beyond what other family members would experience.

After I sensed she was peaceful and resting comfortably later that evening, I kissed her good-bye once again, and said, "I love you." She then did the most astonishing thing. She opened her eyes wide, looked me straight in the eye and winked! I smiled and laughed out loud. I didn't know if she would still be with us when I came to visit tomorrow. That thought did not rest easily with me, though I no longer feared it.

SIXTY-THREE
Loving Caregivers

I dreamt last night that Mom died. When I awakened early this morning, I immediately called Tendercare Cottages to find out whether Mom would be making her final journey down Interstate 90 to our hometown—the funeral home would be coming from Nelson City to retrieve Mom's body, because that's where the funeral and burial would be. Instead, I learned that she lived through the night, and had already had some water to drink this morning.

When I called again a short while later, they said she'd been pretty agitated, moaning and crying out while experiencing more nausea. The caregivers gave her some morphine and she was sleeping soundly. She had stopped breathing several times, only momentarily, and most of her breathing was through her mouth.

After arriving at Tendercare Cottages, I found Mom on the living room couch; she was actually lying in Pat's arms while one of the other daytime caregivers sat on the other side of her. Hospice is a wonderful organization, but it was these women who worked at Tendercare Cottages each and every day who loved and cared for the residents like they were their own parents, who should be recognized and commended. In a sense, I considered these caregivers "family" as they spent so much time with my parents on a daily basis. I was so impressed by these women and the empathy and love they showered on the residents. I will be forever grateful for their loving support during this difficult journey.

I was astonished, yet again, by how much worse Mom looked. Her eyes tended to roll back in her head, and when they did focus, the blue of her irises was covered with a milky glaze. Could she still focus on what was going on around her? I wasn't sure. She was very unresponsive when I talked to her and kissed her hello. She stared at the ceiling and breathed heavily through her mouth. She had some color back in her extremities today, but overall looked more ashen.

It was even more apparent the end was imminent. I felt as if we were standing at the edge of an unknown precipice. This was one tenacious woman, fighting to the end, and not letting go easily, even though we had assured her it was okay to go. Today, I asked her, "Mom, can you please give Grandma a hug when you see her?"

My nieces both called again and asked that I let their grandma know one more time how much they loved her and give her a hug. I could easily do the former, but was almost afraid of breaking her doing the latter, as she was a decidedly delicate, gossamer being.

We laid her back down on the couch, and the caregivers moved aside to let me be near her. Dad rolled up beside us in his wheelchair. He looked down at her, and I was instantly positive that he knew on some level what was happening. I looked at him and tears softly rolled out of the corners of his eyes. I went immediately to him and hugged him tightly, loving him as best I could and he patted my back.

"We'll get through this together, okay, Dad?"

He nodded his head, a silent, "yes."

I squeezed him tighter, and he hugged me back. I felt completely and utterly heartbroken for him. We helped him move closer so he could hold her hand.

"Mom, your husband Harry is holding your hand now."

I held my father's other hand and then grabbed Mom's other hand, forming an unbroken circle, both physically and emotionally. Early scientists and scholars, as well as many spiritual traditions around the world believe there is something intrinsically divine or perfect that can be found in circles, and in this overwhelmingly powerful moment of connection with my parents, I agreed. I was barely holding myself together as tears streamed down my cheeks. I felt richly blessed by this sacred moment.

I don't know if Dad moved into unawareness, was bored, or simply couldn't stand the emotional pain, as he soon let go of our hands and rolled back into his room. Soon he was shouting, "Help, help!" He wanted to go to bed. I wondered if it was to escape reality or if he had forgotten what was happening. Later, he wheeled by me and gave me the biggest smile and completely ignored Mom, so it's impossible to know what was going on inside his brain. However, I was firmly convinced he knew on some level that Mom was dying.

As the afternoon wore on, Mom started to become agitated again, and her feet began twitching, so the caregiver gave her another dose of morphine. They then moved her back onto her bed where she began to sleep peacefully. Meanwhile, Dad finished dinner and wheeled by Mom's door into his room without so much as a second glance. He had forgotten we were there, right next door, as I kept my vigil beside his wife, my mother. Darkness slowly settled around us.

SIXTY-FOUR
And so, it is time ... March 9, 2008

Eventually, I left the facility late last night to attempt sleep, with instructions to the night staff to call me if her condition further deteriorated. And sleep I did, out of sheer emotional exhaustion. With my usual trepidation, I called the facility as soon as I awakened early in the morning. The caregiver answering my call said with a sense of urgency, "She has begun to stop breathing for as long as a minute. You might want to hurry."

What? Why hadn't they called me? What were they waiting for? Not stopping to ask questions, my husband and I hurriedly drove to Tendercare Cottages. Lionel and I went directly to Mom's room, where we found her lying on her mattress on the floor, surrounded by two caregivers and my father. He was staring at her. "How long has she been sick?" he asked me. "What's wrong with her? Does she have something wrong with her stomach?"

Even though I shouldn't have been, I was incredulous. Dementia is a cruel disease. Yesterday, he certainly seemed to be aware, if only for a few minutes. In any case, right now he was fully involved and concerned.

Looking at her, it was apparent that she was struggling to get air. The end was upon us. Tears began their steady descent down my cheeks as I stared at her frail, elfin body.

"I would love for Dad to be able to kiss her and say goodbye. Would that somehow be possible?" I asked Pat through my tears.

"Yes, let's lift her up to him!" she suggested.

Together, Lionel and Pat picked up my featherweight mom, and put her cheek right next to my dad's lips. He puckered up and kissed her many times on the cheek. "Goodbye," he said. "It's okay to go." They laid her back down.

Out of the corner of her eye rolled a single, sparkling tear.

The caregivers then left the four of us alone to spend our last moments together as a family. I sat down beside her on the floor next to her mattress, Lionel in a chair at the head of the mattress, and my father beside me as close as a wheelchair could be.

We spoke softly to her, expressing our love. I measured breaths. At first they were 10 or 12 seconds apart. Next, they were about 30 seconds and then 60 seconds in between the labored mouth breathing. After an interval of 90 seconds, I leaned down and whispered into her ear, "I love you. Safe travels." She breathed her last breath at that precise moment, and then she was gone, gone to join those who went before. I did a strange thing and glanced at the ceiling, just in case I might see her soul floating toward God.

We sat with her a few more moments before Lionel left the room to let the caregivers know she had departed silently, and, I truly think, peacefully.

It didn't occur to us at the time, but in retrospect, Lionel made the comment, "You know, it was a little like attending a birth in that we were timing the breaths much like we time contractions when a baby is born."

There is anticipation, and a metamorphosis beyond our imagination as none can fathom what lies ahead. The newborn no more knows what lies on the other side of the warm, bath-like environment of the womb he is leaving than my mother, or anyone knows of the chrysalis or rebirth into a new dimension into which we all will eventually pass.

EPILOGUE
Several months later ...

It was mid-afternoon on a beautiful cornflower blue-sky summer day when I arrived at Tendercare Cottages to visit my dad. I parked my car in the familiar parking lot where I had parked so many times before. I sighed, stealing a moment before going inside to reflect on all that had happened in the past five years, starting with that pesky computer. It had been a journey of heartbreak and love, of hanging on and letting go. I noted that I had started consistently sleeping uninterrupted through the night again for the first time in years. When people asked me how I was doing, it was with a rather perplexed surprise in my voice when I answered, "I am doing well." I kept waiting for the grief to strike, the tears, the sorrow, and the agony of loss. In complete honesty, so far I had felt mostly relief and realized my stress level had declined significantly.

Should I have guilt that I felt this way? People have told me that this, too, was normal—this feeling of relief and the subsequent guilt it brought. The little girl in me no longer feared my mother's criticisms or tongue lashings of old. It was a feeling of relief on many different levels. Suddenly, without all the stress that came with caring for Mom and her often difficult personality, I was in a much more peaceful place. I also knew that being with her as she departed on her final journey had given me a solid sense of closure in her passing. There was a fulfillment in the letting-go process that I didn't believe I would've gained otherwise. Being present for her departure was truly a blessing for me. After this experience, I now viewed death and dying in a different way. It had taken the scariness factor out of the equation. Granted, I witnessed a very gentle passing, but I sensed that the process was part of the rhythm of the universe. We moved from one dimension to the next at the designated time and place, and we left the same way we arrived—alone, yet not alone. When that time arrived for each of us, I was quite certain guides in many guises, human or otherwise, would surround us for the journey. I knew that what I witnessed in her room on that morning was love in the purest sense. It was my privilege to be there, and the experience would always be remembered in that way.

Dad also seemed to be coping well. In fact, I perceived he'd actually blossomed since Mom passed away. Dad celebrated his 95th birthday a couple of months ago, and if anyone asked him how old he was, he would proudly state, without a moment's hesitation, "I am 95!" He had started asking the caregivers to give him his electric shaver every morning. It seemed nothing short of miraculous that my dad had begun shaving himself, after years of enduring my mother saying she had to shave him, because she felt he wasn't capable. It may take him close to 45 minutes to accomplish the task, but I marveled at how smooth his skin seemed, and I wondered if he didn't have some satisfaction in being able to do *something* for himself once again.

Dad has never asked me about Mom. I contemplated again this afternoon, as I have ruminated on this many times over the past few months, why that was so. It intrigued me, but I have decided, for the moment, to take the Beatles' advice and just "let it be." My dad appeared content with a smile on his face most days when I visited. I reflected on this for a time, and the realization dawned on me that maybe he had also been released, much as I have felt released, from the trauma and anxiety Mom was so capable of causing.

My mind returned to the present moment and I realized my car was becoming excruciatingly hot inside; the time for reflection was over for now. Time to go see what my dad was up to today. I burst through the door of the facility into the cool interior, but didn't see my dad anywhere. I was told he was lying down, which surprised me, and a bit cautiously, I asked, "Is he okay?"

"Yes, he's okay. He just asked to lie down after dinner today to take a break from sitting in his wheelchair." I was reminded again how difficult it must be to be confined to a wheelchair all day long.

I ventured into Dad's room, and found him lying curled up under a blanket on his bed, resting. I was taken slightly aback at how small he looked. His eyes were open.

"Hi! What are you up to?" I asked him.

"Just thinking," he replied.

"What are you thinking?"

"Oh, I don't know, really. Just thinking."

I pursued this line of conversation for a while, but he was unable to verbalize what he was "thinking." I decided to move on to a new subject.

"Would you like to get up?"

"No."

"How are you feeling today?"

"Okay, I guess."

"Do you know who I am?"

"Um, no. Who are you?"

"I'm a relative. Do you know which one?"

"No, can't say as I do."

"Do you have a daughter?" I couldn't help quizzing him.

"Maybe I do."

"Well, it's me, your daughter."

"Yes, I think I do have a daughter," he conceded.

"Yes, you do. That's me. I'm here."

He lay still while I sat next to him, thinking about where to go next with this scintillating conversation. Shortly, the caregiver came into his room to administer his afternoon medication.

"Time to get up. It's four o'clock."

"No. It's too early. I don't want to get up yet."

Recognizing that he thought it was early morning, she replied, "No, it isn't four a.m., it's four p.m."

In a few short and coordinated moves, she sat him up, put his shoes on and transferred him into his wheelchair.

"It's a beautiful, warm sunshiny day today. Let's go for a walk, Dad, okay?" I asked him after she had finished.

"Okay."

I helped him put on a sweater and his green cap, then we were off to walk around the carefully manicured grounds of the facility, noticing the flowers, bushes, trees, and water pond, where we stopped to ponder life together.

"Where are you at now?" he asked, making conversation.

"Well, I live here in Coulson now."

"Where did you come from?"

"I came from my house."

"How was school today?" This came out of nowhere and I wondered once again how my father's brain worked.

"Um, yeah, well, it was fine …" *Was it appropriate to make things up or was it better to be bluntly honest in these cases? I found out with his next question:* "So, what grade are you in now?"

Okay, truth trumps fantasy here ... "Well, actually I am finished with school."

"You are out of high school?" he asked with what I believe was some incredulity. "Are you going to college?"

"I have already finished college. In fact, my three children have also finished college."

"Really?" He contemplated this for a moment before his zinger, "Well, that makes you an old woman then, doesn't it?"

(Chuckling) "Yeah, I guess so, Dad."

I decided to try a new conversational topic. "What can you see?" I asked him.

"Oh, the building we live in," looking in the opposite direction of that building. Then, "Those are really big rocks," as he noticed the rocks surrounding the pond. "That looks like a big pan over there," as he pointed to a large flat rock on the other side of the pond.

We sat in silence a bit longer as I spied an elegant dragonfly with black and white striped wings dancing about from reed to reed in the algae-filled pond. A yellow-tailed bird skittered by and landed next to us in a small Aspen tree, whose emerald-colored leaves fluttered in the breeze. Unfortunately, Dad's eyesight was too poor to see the small and beautiful subtleties of nature like the fluttering dragonflies and birds, or even to distinguish big objects like large, flat boulders. I was reminded to be grateful for my eyesight.

"What do you hear, Dad?"

He thought for a moment before answering, "Birds, I think," as a cricket chirped in the background. We talked about hearing cars moving down the road behind the fenced-in facility. "I didn't know we lived so close to the road," he observed.

What a good idea it had been to go for a walk, as this was one of the longest conversations we had had in a long time. I reminded myself to do this each time I visited, provided he and the weather were both agreeable.

Soon he was ready to move on. "Let's go."

I wheeled him back down the path to the building. "Would you like to go around the path again?"

"No, let's go inside." Off we rolled, on our way to new adventures together.

I was uncertain if I had completely assimilated the fact that Mom was no longer here. And then I thought, *but she was still here!* I found myself buoyed by this idea. Almost on a daily basis, I was reminded of her in so many different ways. She was always such a force in my life that it was impossible *not* to be reminded of her. She was there when I cooked, or cleaned my house, always at the ready with practical suggestions and her answers to living. I carried her with me, and even found myself talking to her now and then. The mother I knew before her illness lived on in my heart and mind. I imagined this to be true for all of our family. There would be chance comments by others or passing thoughts in our own minds, which would remind each of us of Mom. Maybe memories of her would be triggered by the smell of fried chicken or the taste of homemade ice cream. These occurrences would likely assail my family at odd moments of the day or night, and in this happening, our mother/grandmother would be brought to life again in our hearts and we, her legacy, would know her spirit lived on through us all.

AFTERWORD

Dad received the answer to his question, "How long do I have to live," on March 10, 2009, exactly one year and one day after Mom passed away. His departure occurred quickly and peacefully, almost without notice, on a late winter evening, shortly after I received one last good-bye kiss and a softly spoken "love you." In the brief moments of stillness immediately following his passing, I thought to myself how blessed I was to have been present for the deaths of both my parents, helping them pass from this life into the next. As I stepped out into the biting winter air that night, in the midst of my sadness, a half smile crossed my face when I thought that as Dad hadn't shaved for a couple of days at the time of his passing, I was sure Mom met him in the next realm with a shaver in her hand and a twinkle in her eye.

APPENDIX A
More on Plaques and Tangles

All human brains contain amyloid plaques and neuro-fibrillary tangles. What sets apart the brain of someone with Alzheimer's is the gross *amount* of these plaques and tangles. Our brains contain nerve cells called neurons and amyloid plaques are found outside these neurons, while the neuro-fibrillary plaques are found inside.

These plaques and tangles were first identified in an autopsy over 100 years ago, in 1906 in Munich, by German psychiatrist and neuropathologist Alois Alzheimer. Because one of his patients in the asylum where he worked had exhibited "strange" behavior and short-term memory loss, he elected to study the pathology of her brain after she died, and detailed for the first time plaques and tangles found within the brain. He is credited with first describing the disease which bears his name.

Amyloid *plaques* consist primarily of amino acids of a protein called B-amyloid, which is part of a much larger protein called amyloid precursor protein (APP). It is unknown what APP does, but it is made in cells and transported to the cell membrane, where it is later broken down. There are two major pathways involved in the breakdown of AAP, one of which is normal, causing no problems. It is the second pathway that causes the problems, bringing about the changes seen in some dementias, including Alzheimer's disease.

A second major component in the brain of an Alzheimer's patient is neurofibrillary *tangles*. These tangles are composed of a protein called tau protein, which plays a critical role in the structure of neurons. In a person with Alzheimer's disease, tau proteins cause an abnormality through overactive enzymes, which results in the formation of neurofibrillary tangles. These "tangles" cause brain cell death.

The role of amyloid plaques and neurofibrillary tangles in brain function are not fully understood. Ongoing research continues to search for the link between these proteins and the development and progression of Alzheimer's disease.

For More Information :

Alberts, B., Bray, D., Lewis, J., Raff, M.,& Roberts, K. (1989). *Molecular biology of the cell.* 2nd Ed. New York: Garland Publishing.

Alzheimer's Association (2012). *2012 Alzheimer's Disease Facts and Figures.* Retrieved from http://www.alz. org/downloads/facts_figures_2012.pdf.

Del, C. Alonso, A, Zaidi, T., Novak, M., Grundke-Iqbal, I., & Iqbal, K. (2001). Hyperphosphorylation induces self-assembly of τ into tangles of paired helical filaments/straight filaments. *Proceedings of the National Academy of Science, 98*(12), 6923-6928.

Goedert, M., Spillantini, M.G. (2006). *Science, 314* (5800), 777-781.

Goetz, C.G. (2003). *Textbook of clinical neurology,* 2nd Ed. Philadelphia: Saunders Publishing.

Kenard, C. (2005). *Explanations on plaques and tangles from the Alzheimer's brain.* Retrieved from: About. com Health's Disease and Condition content is reviewed by Suman Jayadev, MD

Mayeux, R., Denaro, J., Hemenegildo, N., Marder, K., Tang, M.X., Cote, L.J., & Stern, A. (1992). A population-based investigation of Parkinson's disease with and without dementia. Relationship to age and gender. *Archives of Neurology, 49*(5), 492-297.

Murat, E. (2004). Rivastigmine for dementia associated with Parkinson's Disease, *New England Journal of Medicine, 351,* 2509-2518.

Pearson, H.A., & Peers C. (2006). Physiological roles for amyloid β peptides. *Journal of Physiology, 575*(1), 5-10.

Turner, P,R., O'Connor, K., Tate, W.P., & Abraham, W.C. (2003). Roles of amyloid precursor protein and its fragments in regulating neural activity plasticity, and memory. *Progress in Neurobiology, 70*(1),1-32.

Walsh, D.M., Klyubin, I., Fadeeva, J.V., Rowan, M.J., & Selkoe, D.J. (2002). The role of cell-derived oligomers of Aβ in Alzheimer's disease and avenues for therapeutic intervention. *Biochemical Society Transactions, 30*(4), 552-557.

APPENDIX B
Understanding the Difference between Alzheimer's Disease and Dementia

There is an extremely helpful booklet entitled *My Past is Now My Future; A Practical Guide to Dementia Possible Care*, co-authored by Larry Butler, MS, OTR, and Kari Brizendine, PT, both therapists who work with dementia patients. They state that dementia is a "global term" for cognitive and memory function loss, meaning that Alzheimer's disease is only one of around 70 different types of dementia. A diagnosis of dementia means that at least two brain spheres are impaired. These spheres include memory, orientation, language, attention, perception, and "the ability to carry out purposeful tasks." Fifty percent of diagnosed irreversible dementia is called Alzheimer's disease, making it by far the most commonly diagnosed type of dementia. A "true" diagnosis of Alzheimer's is made only after doing an autopsy of the Alzheimer patient's brain, which will show a smaller brain filled with plaques and tangles.

APPENDIX C

The Mini Mental State Examination (MMSE) test screens for the presence of cognitive impairment in a number of different areas. Cognition is defined as "mental activity, such as memory, thinking, attention, reasoning, decision making, and dealing with concepts." The test, which is quick and easily administered, was developed in the 1970s by Dr. Marshall Folstein, and is used widely in both the U.S. and the U.K.

The patient undergoing examination is asked a series of questions, with points assigned to each correct answer. The maximum score is 30 points; people with dementia/Alzheimer's generally score less than 26 points.

Questions are divided into different sections.

1. Orientation (Up to 10 points): this section tests a patient's awareness of location and date.

2. Memory (up to 6 points): this section tests recall ability by asking patients to remember three words, which the patient will be asked to provide from memory later in the test. If he or she is able to recall the list on both occasions, he/she is awarded 6 points (3 points for each incidence).

3. Attention and Calculation (up to 5 points): this section tests the person's ability to concentrate. She may be asked to subtract, for example, 7 from 100, and continue going backwards five times. Another way to test this is to have him/her or her spell a word backwards. He/she might be asked to do both; the best score would be used.

4. Language, Writing and Drawing (up to 9 points): this section tests both written and spoken language, as well as the ability to write, copy, and remember named objects. The person is shown an item and must correctly identify it. Next he/she is asked to repeat a sentence. Lastly, he/she is asked to write a sentence and also to copy a figure or shape on a piece of paper.

The scores are added up to give a result of the MMSE.

Score results of the MMSE indicates the stage of Alzheimer's disease as follows:

Scores indicating dementia:
- Scores of 27 and above are considered normal
- Scores of 23 to 26 indicate a borderline condition
- Scores of 22 and below are abnormal

Scores indicating Alzheimer's disease:
- Scores of 20 to 26 suggest mild Alzheimer's disease
- Scores of 10 to 19 show moderate Alzheimer's disease
- Scores below 10 indicate severe Alzheimer's disease

On average, people with Alzheimer's disease that do not receive treatment (i.e., medications) lose 2 to 4 points on the MMSE each year.

Folstein, M. F., Folstein, S. E., & McHugh, P. (1975). A practical method for grading the cognitive state of patients for the clinician. *Journal of Psychiatric Research, 12*(3), 189-198.

APPENDIX D

The Alzheimer's Association Montana newsletter published a list that I found extremely helpful along our journey. My only problem was "remembering" to follow it.

The Dos and Don'ts:

Don't reason

Don't argue

Don't confront

Don't remind them they forget

Don't question recent memory

Don't take it personally

Do give short, one-sentence explanations

Do allow plenty of time for comprehension, and then triple it

Do repeat instructions of sentences exactly the same way

Do eliminate "but" from your vocabulary, substitute "nevertheless"

Do avoid insistence—try again later

Do agree with them or distract them to a different subject or activity

Do accept the blame when something's wrong (even if it's a fantasy)

Do leave the room, if necessary, to avoid confrontation

Do respond to the feelings rather than the words

Do be patient and cheerful and reassuring

Do go with the flow

Do practice 100 percent forgiveness—memory loss progresses daily

Be generous. Be gracious. Okay?

Reprinted with permission.

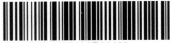

Made in the USA
Columbia, SC
25 July 2018